a whole new normal

a whole new normal

An Acoustic Neuroma Journey

marla bronstein

S.H. Publishing

Library of Congress No. 2013913901
ISBN: 9780615852133

Published 2013
Printed in the United States of America.

For information www.awholenewnormal.com

To my mother, who gave me life, and gave her life for me.

CONTENTS

INTRODUCTION

My doctor's nurse calls me on the phone, and nonchalantly tells me I have a life-threatening condition. A brain tumor.

Now what?

It was the first of a thousand other questions I would find myself faced with in the days, weeks and months ahead. Which symptoms are worse? Which doctor should I consult with? Which one should I trust? Which course of treatment is best?

Will I survive?

In this book, I am sharing my own personal questions and my own answers. Mine are only mine. I am not saying my answers are the answers you should come up with.

Except the answer to this one:

Will things ever be normal again?

The answer is yes. For everyone. There will be a whole new normal.

Going at a rate of 150 miles per hour, with ten balls in the air and multiple projects going every day, my calendar is scheduled out weeks in advance, weekends are booked months out. This is how I have lived since my freshman year of college. Back then, I'd go to work at the school radio station at 6:00 AM, go to my first class at 9:00 AM, work in the dorm mail room in the afternoon, and study at the campus library at night; every minute of the day was accounted for. Fast forward thirty years, and I'm a married working mother of two who's involved in the community and who does volunteer work. I have no time to read a book, (much less, write one), do a craft project for fun, or, God forbid, die.

Chapter 1. SYMPTOMS

In the spring of 1982, I was twenty-five, living in Long Beach. I had just been let go from a job that I didn't love, was recovering emotionally from a broken engagement from a guy my parents didn't love, and was recovering physically and financially from a major car accident that was not my fault. This particular morning, I walked down to the beach to contemplate my future while staring out at the Pacific Ocean. I was attempting to get grounded in the present so I could figure out my future. I closed my eyes and took a deep relaxing breath. Suddenly, I experienced a sharp piercing pain in my left ear that jerked me to attention. The pain came in waves, causing me to spasm. I'm not sure how long it lasted, an hour maybe? A few measured breaths made it subside. I attributed it to stress, and went home, ignoring the message I was getting from my head.

The pain returned and ceased intermittently for a few days, and then it completely stopped just as suddenly. As a kid, I had grown up with ear infections—I had them many times in both ears. So I went to the doctor, thinking it might be yet another ear infection. But they looked in my ear, and found nothing unusual.

Ten years later, in the spring of 1992, I was married to Ken. We had moved to Bellingham with our two year old daughter

Zoe, and I was 6 months pregnant with our second child. The sharp pain returned after years of absence, as suddenly as it had disappeared. By then I had also noticed a hearing issue in my left ear; sounds were a little muffled. Again, I went to the doctor to check for an ear infection. Again, they looked in my ear, and found nothing unusual.

For the next sixteen years, I learned to live with decreased hearing, intermittent dizziness, and headaches. In all that time, I never asked the doctor for a hearing test. I just figured it was all in my head.

Little did I know, it really was.

I'm the mom. I'm the caretaker. I'm the multi-tasker. I figure things out, and I help other people figure things out. I don't know everything, but I know how to find things. If you ask me a question or pose me a problem, I'll do my very best to help you figure out the answer. If you're not feeling well, I'll make sure you eat right, make sure you drink your water, and even drive you to the doctor if you need me to.

But me? I can take care of myself. I don't need anyone's help—or so at least that's what I thought. I go to the doctor every year for the annual "poke and grope," as my friend Jan calls it. I get my eyes checked regularly, but not my hearing. It's just not one of the things they regularly check when you're an adult, unless you ask.

In the fall of 2008, the hearing in my left ear had become so distorted that I could not distinguish voices on the telephone at work. And a new symptom, a constant intense ringing and humming. My ear didn't hurt, so I was sure it wasn't an infection. I wrote it off to residual symptoms of a cold or something, and I let it just work itself out for a few weeks. But the problems persisted for a month. I finally called my doctor.

By the time I sought out medical attention for my hearing issue, I had changed primary care physicians twice since that appointment sixteen years earlier. I found Ann's practice based upon a recommendation by a massage therapist when my son was about two years old. Ann was different. She and the entire staff really listened to me and explored my medical symptoms and concerns without making me feel like I was a hypochondriac. I asked her to give me a referral to a local ENT—an ear, nose, and throat specialist— who had successfully treated and cured both my son and my husband for ear problems in the past. She gave me the referral to be used in late December, with the understanding that if my symptoms subsided by then, I'd cancel the appointment.

I believe in both Western medicine and alternative medicine, so in early December, I saw my chiropractor and my acupuncturist. My chiropractor said I had a systemic yeast infection, and he recommended a Candida diet for six months which strictly limited my sugar, carb and vegetable intake. I basically lived on rice cakes and almond butter. I was cracked, adjusted, lasered, chanted to, and given lots of vitamins and herbs. At the same time, I went to my acupuncturist Paula who poked me in my head, my hands, my face, and my feet.

By the middle of the month, my hearing problems had not subsided, so at the end of the month, as planned, I finally had my appointment with the ENT.

After looking in my ear, seeing nothing unusual, and finally doing a hearing test, he told me I had some hearing loss (duh!), gave me a prescription for an antibiotic, and asked me to come back in three or four months if I wasn't better. He said there might be a "tumor or something", but not to worry and he'd send me for an MRI if it wasn't better by mid-winter. In March, I was back at the same ENT. I had my hearing tested again. The ringing, distortion and muffled hearing hadn't cleared up. I asked if I could be scheduled for that MRI he'd mentioned back in December. Again he said I should wait three or four more months for the MRI. To this day, I don't know why he never sent me for an MRI.

Over the course of the next three months, I saw my chiropractor twelve times. I had a total of three acupuncture treatments to clear up head and sinus congestion, and I bought lots of herbal stuff to spray, swallow and snort.. I generally felt better—the congestion was less substantive, but the treatments and the herbs made no difference in my hearing or the ringing in my ear.

In early June, the frustration finally got to me. I knew I'd have to go out of town to see a different ENT—I live in Bellingham, outside of Seattle, and the ENT I was seeing was the only practice in town. I called my primary care doctor again and asked for a referral to a different ENT practice, explaining mine would not give me a referral for the MRI. Instead of sending me to another specialist, however, my hero doc scheduled me for an MRI the very next week!

I went in on the morning of June 10, 2009. It was my husband's birthday. The test itself went well. Being inside the MRI machine is sort of like being in a tanning booth with more clothes, less lights and no quick exit. I just kept my eyes closed. I had one copy of the MRI sent to Ann, and ordered one for myself. I also had one sent to the ENT, (who I will refer to from here on out as Dr. Death--I probably shouldn't call him that since I am technically still alive. But I could/would not have been.) That same afternoon, my doctor's nurse called me to talk about the results. (It's never a good sign when your doctor's office calls you the afternoon of a lab test. I know that from past experience.)

The nurse started off by telling me I had something called an "acoustic neuroma, also called a vestibular schwannoma." She told me that it was kind of rare, that it was benign, it was life threatening, and that she wanted to schedule an appointment for the next day for me to come in with my husband and talk to my doctor about the results.

I wrote down acoustic neuroma, and as soon as I hung up the phone, I looked it up on the Internet. The photos, videos, and websites that came up scared the ever-living bajeebes out of me. By the time I saw my doctor the next day, she told me what I had already learned: that the acoustic neuroma was a tumor on my eighth auditory nerve—causing the ringing, deafness, and dizziness—and that it might need to come out, but that I definitely needed to see a neurosurgeon.

So began a series of referrals to specialists just to figure out what was in my head. My doc's poor referral administrator was so patient with me.

Referral 1 was to a local neurosurgeon. When I called to see the specific doctor named, the receptionist told me that he had no appointments available for two months. When she offered another doctor in the practice, I asked if that other doctor was familiar with my diagnosis. The receptionist told me that they had hardly ever treated that condition in their office. I said thanks anyway, never mind, and got a new referral.

Referral 2 was a specialist neurosurgeon in Seattle. His online bio was minimal. As luck would have it, Ken and I have a friend who is also a physician in Seattle. We called him to get the 411 on this neurosurgeon, and our friend said he had never heard of him. He did have a name of a specialist otolaryngologist (try saying that three times fast!) also in Seattle, to suggest, who became Referral 3.

The last Friday in June, Ken and I drove the 90 mile trip to Seattle and spent two hours planning my future with a man I had never met before. Dr. Referral 3 worked out of a well-respected teaching hospital, and showed up for my first appointment with a crew of students in tow. He spent more time addressing them than talking to me. While I appreciated his knowledge, in the long run, I felt I needed more connection to the person I was going to trust my life and health with. Nevertheless, here is what I can tell you I know by the end of this part of the process:

- Yes, there is a tumor.
- No, it is not cancer.
- Yes, I will lose all the hearing in my left ear.
- No, the ringing in my left ear will probably not go away.
- Yes, there is a slight chance I will have nerve damage in my face.
- No, it does not need to come out today, this week, or this month.

- Yes, they will have to cut the nerve in my ear that helps with balance.
- No, I won't be able to go for a long walk right away.
- Yes, I will be able to drink adult beverages shortly after surgery.
- No, I will not be able to drive for a few months.
- Yes, it needs to come out. If I do not get it removed, it could continue to grow, push on my brain stem, stop me from breathing and I could die.

This was June. I had stuff on my calendar through December.

You know that John Lennon saying, "Life is what happens to you while you are busy making other plans"? Maybe that explains why I've always done a million things at once. I knew maybe intuitively, it would all catch up eventually. I have piles of books and projects saved "for when I can't get up and move, or if I ever break a leg." Here was that opportunity, and I bet it had been with me for a long time.

I wanted/needed to get all the information, form a plan of attack, and understand the prognosis in order to keep my family, especially my children, from worrying. I didn't want anyone to worry. If I could have gotten it taken care of without saying anything to anyone, I would have.

Ken and I sat down that night at the end of June, after I saw the last neurosurgeon, and tried to explain to our kids what we knew and what we didn't know. We tried to calm their fears; we told them that I was going to be around for a while and that everything would be going back to normal. We told them we weren't sure how or when that would happen, and we told them we didn't know what "normal" was going to look like.

So began my journey of a whole new normal. I started an online journal to communicate to my network of family and friends without having to repeat the same story over and over. Along with some of the entries that follow are a fraction of the thousands of responses from family, friends, and strangers-now-friends that lifted me when I was low and carried me through. These comments have been edited for space only.

Chapter 2. DEALING WITH THE DIAGNOSIS

There are two ways to die. Fast, like a heart attack or as a result of an accident. The people who are left to pick up the pieces can barely function. I think this is because there is so much guilt over things left unsaid and the special moments missed.

Or they die slowly, with long-lasting and painful events (emotional and/or physical) from cancer or Alzheimer's or surgery complications. All goodbyes are said; all last kisses are shared. Those left want the dying person to be "let go" to not have to endure one more day of living hell. But after the person dies, there is so much guilt about feeling "relief" that it is over. It's a lose-lose.

I knew I wasn't going to die … well, that's not true. No one gets out of here alive. I just started to feel a little less sure that I had a long life ahead.

By this time, I had started telling more people in my inner and outer circles about my diagnosis. I had shared the online blog through Facebook and email. It was also searchable, which meant anyone in the world who searched for "acoustic neuroma" within the journal site could find it and read it. When friends (and sometimes strangers) commented on my journal posts, I felt like we were having a conversation. Even though I'm normally (hah!) a private person who tries really hard to not complain about stuff to friends, much less strangers, it made me feel very supported. I never commented after someone else did (except once.) I'm including some comments as they were responses to specific journal posts because they made me think, laugh, or just because their comment added a bit to what I had posted. I've added my responses here where I feel like I needed to add something.

December 8, 2009: He said, "See ya!"

I had not seen Dr. Death professionally since March of 2009. Even after sending the results of the initial MRI in June, I heard nothing from him.

A lot of people I knew died during that first six months of my diagnosis. Some were old. Some were not. Some of the younger ones were sick a long time. Some of them were sick for such a short time, I had a hard time believing they were really gone. I would fantasize about my funeral, if I had one, who would come, what kind of music they would play ...

It was September, and I was just leaving the memorial for an amazing woman who had died slowly; she had been sick for years. She was lovely and loved. It was a very moving service. As I left the mortuary, there was Dr. Death, walking toward me—well, in my direction anyway. I was standing by the parking lot. Our eyes met. He said nothing ... and then, there it was ... a smile and a nod.

A SMILE AND A NOD??

I was expecting a little more than that. Okay, so maybe a funeral was not the time or place to talk to me about my diagnosis. I'll give him that. It's been months since then. I have barely given him a second thought.

But today I was having lunch with my friend Mish. As our food is being served, who should walk in and sit down at the table right in my line of sight? Bingo. Dr. Death. He says hi, I say hi. We go back to eating our lunches. Sort of. I take a moment to retrain myself to breathe again.

Thank the universe Mish is there to talk me down. The two of us have a very pleasant lunch, in spite of everything, although

I am somewhat distracted by the fact that I know I have to say something to him before I leave the restaurant. Right?

We are minutes from leaving, and I tell her I am ready, I am going to say something, but that I'll wait until she leaves so I don't embarrass her. But without warning, Dr. Death and his lunch companion stand up, toss their trash, and exit the restaurant. I watch them leave, and then, as if it is an afterthought, Dr. Death pokes his head back around the door and looks at me, gives me an enormous grin, and says "See ya!" And that's it. He's gone.

Nothing. Not one word about my tumor, after fifteen years of being our family's "go-to" ENT, after all of my hearing tests, after getting a copy of my MRI last summer. Nothing.

Mish and I look at each other and burst out laughing. Not because it was funny. Because it was completely ridiculous. I could not believe it! I shook my head, realizing I'd lost my opportunity for closure. But my dear sweet brilliant friend asked me what I would have said. Here it is:

"I am sad and disappointed in you as a health-care professional. You are not the person I thought you were. I trusted the health of my family to you for over fifteen years. You operated on my son twice. When I came to you for help, I completely trusted you and your expertise. When I asked for diagnostic testing for myself, you refused twice.

"I had to go elsewhere to have the test that showed I have a life-threatening condition. You received a copy of the MRI. And you never contacted me. And today, not a 'How are you? How is the family?' I would have expected nothing more."

Done and done. Now that I've said these things—though only to Mish—I feel like he owes me nothing. That's closure.

COMMENTS

When I first moved to Bellingham, I met Caryn while she was a practicing free-spirit musician and craft-person. Since then, she has "settled down" to be a piano and guitar teacher. She oozes love and her smile can light up a room.

CARYN said: Had you not been so determined you could still be in limbo. It's a good example for the rest of us concerning how much our health care is really in our own hands. (Doctors can't always be trusted to diagnose our problems or to even care about us).

My response: I always knew I had to advocate for myself. I never thought it would save my life. I never wanted to be one of those patients who was always complaining. And after all those times I was told my ear pain was "nothing" I was shocked to find out it really was "something."

Ann and I met when our daughters were freshmen in the same high school. She and I could not have been more different politically or in our religious beliefs. Because of our similarities in the things that really mattered, mutual respect, love of family and friends and true loyalty, she and I became and remain to this day, fast and forever friends.

ANN said: Here is what I can say, "He doesn't know you, at all, does he." You will get the last word, eventually.

My response: I'd really like him to have the last word. I'd like it to be "sorry."

Every year since 1998, without fail, Ken and I have hosted a community Chanukah party. We'd make a big batch of potato latkes and invite all our friends and ask them to bring side dishes. At seven thirty, we'd light candles and tell the story of Chanukah. The younger kids would exchange homemade gifts. While Ken and the kids could invite anyone they wanted, it was really my party, as I did most of the prep work. (Confession: Ken did most of the post-party cleaning.) If you were invited once, you were invited forever. The parties got bigger every year, and we topped one hundred guests for the first time (but not the last time) in 2006! I knew that by 2011, both kids would "age out" and be off to various colleges, living out of the area. Not knowing what the outcome of my treatment decision would be, I told Ken and the kids that December 2009 might be our last Chanukah party.

December 18, 2009: It's not cancer, so why am I not completely relieved?

I waited—okay, procrastinated—making a decision about surgery for about six months after my diagnosis. The neurosurgeon in Seattle had assured me that waiting six months was not going to kill me. It wasn't like living with a time bomb. The tumor was slow growing. It wouldn't "harden" in its spot. I was relieved to know that I had some time to think it over. Deciding to wait the six months to schedule surgery until after the Chanukah party gave me a lot of time to read, research, study, and worry. Oh, and how I worried myself into a tizzy—sometimes into the occasional panic attack. To distract myself, I created a bucket list. I traveled a bit; I visited long-lost friends and relatives in New York, Chicago, and Los Angeles, just in case it turned out I couldn't travel for a while, or died on the table. I performed my first wedding that summer using the ordination I got online about ten years earlier. I was in a show at the local community theatre.

I kept busy by taking on new tasks, most of them short-term. I didn't make any commitments for the New Year, I knew I'd have to make a major decision after the Chanukah party and so I kept my calendar open.

Also during those six months, I continued to receive acupuncture. I was feeling dizzy and tired and spacey, so I did a forty-day toxic cleanse. I ate lots of fruits and vegetables, and for eight of those forty days, I ate only a puree of steamed green beans, zucchini (fresh from my friend Jill's garden), and celery. (My son said the concoction smelled like vegetable fart, though he graciously held that opinion in until after I was done with that part of the cleanse.) I didn't feel deprived at all during the entire cleanse, and I felt a lot better afterward.

After that first perusal of the internet after my diagnosis, I did a lot more online research on my tumor. I joined online acoustic neuroma forums in Canada and the US. I joined acoustic neuroma Facebook groups. I was able to "chat" with other folks all over the world who had this condition. There were a lot of us. There were a dozen that I know of in my county of just over two hundred thousand people. I wonder how many go undiagnosed? If I hadn't pushed my doc, I'd still be happily oblivious. (No, that's not true; I'd probably be dead.)

Most of the people I met on line and in town were post-surgical. It was really challenging to find people who had this tumor who were in my same position of early diagnosis, denial and delaying the inevitable. It was equally difficult to find information and guidance to help me figure out what to do.

As it turned out, there were two national acoustic neuroma conferences the summer I was diagnosed. One was going to be in Chicago, the other in Vancouver, Canada. Ironically, before I even knew about the conference there, I had scheduled a trip to Chicago a few weeks before the conference dates. I didn't want to (and couldn't afford to) head back to Chicago again that summer. I met a woman named Adrienne in the acoustic neuroma forum. She lived just across the Canadian border from me. She told me she'd be at the Vancouver conference. We agreed to look for each other.

In September 2009, I drove 60 miles to the Vancouver conference, and I'll tell you, walking in that door was REALLY hard. I stood outside the entry door looking in, the first people I saw were three women who had suffered facial nerve damage. When I saw them, I felt lightheaded. I sort of freaked out. I wanted to turn to leave, to go home where it was safe and I knew/saw nothing, but it was too late. I had to know. I had to see what the future possibly held for me. If my life was going to be this, I had to face it.

The women were very nice and welcomed me graciously. As it turned out, I was the only person they expected to have at the conference from the States. I decided to sit at a table toward the front of the room so I wouldn't feel so compelled to look at anyone other than the speakers on the panel. The symposium was held in a conference room with about ten round tables that sat eight each. Some other folks eventually joined me—and they were nice; everyone was nice. The docs talked one at a time—the surgeon, the neurologist, the radiologist. I asked them all a million questions. They patiently answered them all. During the break, I had the nerve to speak to one doctor directly. It was the first time I was able to get recommendations for treatment from physicians who had nothing to gain, since there was no way they could operate on me.

The turning point for me was midday when a little lady—she was maybe five foot one—with severe facial nerve damage talked about her AN journey. She was diagnosed as a very young woman, when she was a new mother. When she talked about what she looks like now, versus who she is and how she feels on the inside, I could not stop crying. I cried a lot that day, I think I was the only one crying. Maybe not.

Out of the forty or so people there that day who had had surgery, most of them had some level of facial nerve damage. And they didn't walk around moping or feeling sorry for themselves. They found their support group, and they lived their lives. There were people there who I thought were like me, pre-surgery, or "watch and wait" those who were getting annual or semi-annual MRIs to see if their tumor was growing. And then there were these two beautiful women. Neither had any facial nerve damage, and I could not for the life of me guess why they were there. Then one got up and spoke—she was on the national executive board. It turned out that both women had had the surgery. One of them, Cheryl, had her surgery three years earlier, and the other, turned out to be Adrienne, my on-line friend, and she had just been operated on in the past four months! Both had had their surgeries done by one of the doctors at the conference. Except for their strategic seating placement (they chose seats in order to put their best ear forward), I would never have guessed it.

I learned a lot that day:

- Doctors in Canada get paid regardless of the kind of treatment prescribed to a patient, so if the surgery isn't going to immediately save your life, and it's most likely not going to make symptoms better, they will opt to make the patient wait as long as possible for treatment, holding that spot open for someone in way worse shape.

- Tumors can grow without a change in symptoms

- Symptoms can change without tumor growth.

- It is common for MRIs to be misread. Sometimes these errors can cause tumors to look up to 0.2 millimeters bigger or smaller than they really are.

- Tumors will eventually stop growing. They cannot, however, determine when they will stop, and they will not guarantee that they won't grow again.

I talked to the surgeon who operated on Adrienne and Cheryl. He recommended a doctor for me to consult with in Seattle who worked out of Virginia Mason hospital. He also agreed to compare my MRI results from the June test with the one I had yet to schedule for December. He said based upon the tumor's size and location, if there was any change noticeable between the two MRIs, he would make a recommendation for me to either go ahead and schedule surgery or watch and wait based upon what he would tell me if I were actually his patient. So at the end of the day, I had made new friends and gotten more information about the tumors, surgical options, and post surgery outcomes. I was a little relieved and extremely exhausted.

A month later, an AN support group was meeting south of Tacoma where I met two people who had had the surgery done by the SAME doctor recommended to me by the surgeon in

Vancouver. Both of them had shown good results as well! Huz-zah!! This was the first time I was able to feel hopeful since my diagnosis!

October, November and the first part of December flew by. One week after the Chanukah party, I headed to my second MRI This test that would tell me if the tumor had grown, stayed the same size, or (oh please oh please oh please) gotten smaller. In all the reading I'd done up to this point, I'd never heard of an Acoustic Neuroma getting smaller, but I was pray-ing it might be possible.

The second MRI was more emotionally difficult than the first. I'm not claustrophobic, but I just could not stop the tears the whole time I was there. I know there are a lot of people that hate the MRI machine because it is so small and containing. I just close my eyes and dream of the beach. A really noisy, airless beach. It works.

Anyway, I didn't want bad news, I wanted the tumor to fear me and shrink. Not that spontaneous shrinking was a possibil-ity. I had copies of this second MRI sent to Ann, the doctor in Canada, and again to the ENT I had seen earlier in the year.

That afternoon, my doctor's office called to tell me the ra-diologist recorded a "0.1 to 0.2 millimeter growth" from the last MRI. (Note to all health care physicians: When you call your patients on their cell phones, make sure they are in a safe place before you give them any bad news. I was DRIVING for God's sake!!)

After a few hours of panic and hysterics, I remembered what I'd learned about how common it is for MRIs to be misread, so I decided that the tumor's growth was actually a misread and that in fact there had been no change. I proceeded to celebrate this lack of growth by getting my drunk on that night.

On December 16, I received a call from the surgeon in Can-ada. He had reviewed both MRIs and he confirmed what I had most feared … Because the tumor was growing, I could not put off the inevitable surgery. It was a short phone call, but it put me on a track I had been circling and avoiding for six months.

The next day, I had my first consultation appointment with the recommended surgeon in Seattle.

———

One of the things I started doing right away after my diagnosis, beyond continuing chiropractic treatment, acupuncture, and a change of diet, was researching what I called "paths to recovery." I figured the doctors would do their work. I'd have to meet them halfway, and I planned to be in my best shape physically. I knew there would be an emotional component to my preparation as well. I gathered my "support team" consisting at the beginning of only my closest family and friends and grew exponentially. I've never been into the culture of chanting, mantras, crystals, and visualization, but since my tumor and I were intimately connected, I felt like I needed to name it. I'm not sure why I thought the tumor deserved a male name, but I named him "Norman the Neuroma." This was a step up from "Timmy the Tumor" because Timmy was too young and innocent a name for him. Norman, like Norman Bates from Psycho, was insane and needed to be stopped.

December 20, 2009: Becoming mere mortal

I met with Douglas Backous, the doctor recommended to me by his peers and his patients, my surgeon of choice, for the first time on December 17 at Virginia Mason Hospital in Seattle. When he opened the door to the exam room, the light was so bright behind him, it was as if he was glowing with a heaven-like aura. He walked in, and I noticed a Superman twinkle in his eye and dimple in his chin. I swear I heard angels sing. Maybe that was the tinnitus (the technical term for a ringing in the ear) ... but it didn't matter. I liked him immediately. He was very present and attentive. Since then, my friends and family have been referring to him (behind his back) as Dr. Superman.

He also was the only doctor who thought there was a chance, albeit slight, that he could save some of the residual hearing in my left ear. My potentially being completely deaf or hard of hearing would only be a challenge for my non-signing hearing friends. I had been working as a sign language interpreter for the hearing impaired for years. My deaf friends were ready for me.

I also met with Dr. Farrokh Farrokhi, the neurosurgeon that Dr. Superman teams with. The surgery I planned to have was a retrosigmoid craniotomy, in which Dr. Farrokhi would open my head, Dr. Backous would mess with (the technical term) the tumor at the ear canal from behind my brain while Dr. Farrokhi monitored the nerves, and then Dr. Farrokhi would do more detail work with the facial nerve before he closed me up. They'd have to move my brain out of the way to get to the neuroma. It sounded like I was going to be a little more scrambled than usual, but Dr. Superman assured me that the surgery, recovery, and success rate were quite the same as the other procedure options.

My vanity was in full force here, and I continued to be freaked out about my facial nerve, but the fear came in waves. I tried to stay focused on the recovery of my energy level. I knew I would be able to walk and talk, but I was not sure how long it would take me to be able to do both at the same time. Would I be able to adjust and fly to New York for a long weekend? Drive to Portland for the day? Get up and walk the lake, go to work, come home, cook dinner, and do laundry? And if not, how long would it take before I could? Not one my care providers had these answers, and I found that to be the most frustrating of all. With all the power and people using the Internet, I would think someone out there would have, should have, could have known to help put my mind at ease.

It's the not knowing that's the worst. I wanted all my questions answered NOW!

COMMENTS

Jill is my zucchini supplier and occasional acupuncturist and is very much the supportive all-over healer!

JILL said: So glad you have a surgeon with the right attitude.

Virginia's comments are always very calming:

VIRGINIA said: Strength, peaceful moments, and courage your way.

Ro's personal health experience (surgery/complications/recovery) was one of the reasons I knew I had to be ready for any circumstance and situation. She continues to be one of my greatest emotional supporters.

RO said: From my experience, being held in the thoughts of a loving community really does see one through the dark nights.

December 23, 2009: I don't even know what I don't know

Now I know the When (February 10, 2010) and the Why (the tumor is definitely still growing) and the How (retrosigmoid, through the back of my head) and the Where (Virginia Mason in Seattle) and the Who (Doug Backous, otolaryngologist, and Farrokh Farrokhi, neurosurgeon.)

The many questions remaining all start with "What."

Presurgery: What should I do to get ready? What should I eat? What foods/drugs/vitamins should I avoid? What paperwork do I need to have completed? What if I don't get enough sleep between now and February 10? What should I do about expectations to return to work?

And post surgery: What will I be like when I first wake up from surgery? What will I be like a week later, a month later, a year later? What will I need as far as caregiving? What will I want to eat? What will I be able to do? What shouldn't I do?

Getting the answers to these questions should keep me busy for the next forty-nine days. My friends and care providers are so patient with me as I try to take better care of myself. Not just in what I eat and drink, but in my emotional health as well. I am very protective of my time, and yet I try to make time for everyone who is important to me. You know the songs "Live Like You Were Dying," by Tim McGraw and "The Climb," by Miley Cyrus? (You would think I'm a country-music fan, but I'm not.) Both are popular and seem to be playing on the radio every time I turn it on. I have them on my iPod also. These are my grounding songs because they make me take stock of where I am in the moment, and they help me balance what I can give with what I need to get in that moment.

By the way, I made a new AN-survivor friend today. His name is Adam. He found me online.

COMMENTS

Margaret and her husband Jay were at our first Chanuka party, and have attended almost every one since. She is a librarian and works for our local newspaper. From one extreme of literature to another.

MARGARET said: Just be aware that the circle of love of your friends is a mighty powerful thing.

MY response: Always important to remember.

I include this long message from Adam because his detail of his post-surgical experience was the first I had seen that explained all of the stuff I'd wake up with. His matter-of-fact, not-complaining facts were refreshing. We became surgery buddies after this.

ADAM said: Hi Marla, I found your page when searching for other patients with vestibular schwannomas. I know exactly what you're going through—I had a retrosigmoid craniotomy on 11/18/09. In fact, I'll probably be having another one around the same time as yours. My first craniotomy was to do a biopsy to find out what it is and whether or not it is malignant. My second one will be to go back in and remove some of it to decompress my brainstem.

As far as what to expect after surgery, some of it is just recovering from general anesthesia, some of it is recovering from having your head opened and cerebellum retracted, and the rest of it will depend on whether or not you have any nerves damaged during surgery. Since mine was a biopsy, my surgeon was very conservative and removed a small sample, so I had no nerve damage whatsoever. They awakened me in the OR after my surgery, and I drifted in and out of consciousness as they wheeled me into the ICU. I spent the rest of the day and that night in the Neurological ICU. I had an oxygen mask, countless electrodes monitoring my heart, a urinary catheter, a regular IV line, a second sewn-in IV line, and a central line in a vein in my upper chest (everything but the regular IV line was put in after I was under anesthesia). My nurse checked on me constantly, checking my temperature and monitoring what was on all the equipment that was attached to me. I was in quite a bit of pain and had pretty bad nausea. They gave me morphine for pain and anti-nausea medicine. I actually found that Lortab was much more effective at managing my pain than morphine, so that's what I took once I could drink water the first night.

The morning after my surgery, they moved me to a regular room. I continued to receive nausea meds, pain meds, steroids, and muscle relaxers. The muscle relaxers help a little with the pain from the surgeon cutting through the muscles behind your ear. They got me out of bed about thirty hours after my surgery, and I walked up and down the hall (very softly). That evening I tried to eat some, but my appetite was just not back yet. Also, salty foods tasted extremely salty and sweet foods tasted extremely sweet for a few days (it progressively got better).

They let me go home on Saturday (surgery was Wednesday). The car ride home was pretty brutal—I felt every little bump, so you may want to consider the car you ride home in.

One week after surgery, I was able to give my head a good wash—it was covered in Betadine. I was feeling somewhat better by then, but it still hurt to ride in the car, I tired easily, and it hurt to walk unless I stepped softly. I found myself waking up in pain during the middle of the night for a couple of weeks. After the first two weeks went by, my recovery kind of plateaued until I was about four weeks post-op. At that point I kind of spontaneously got much better, so don't get discouraged if you feel like you're not improving. I couldn't drive until four weeks post-op—mostly because my neck was stiff (I'm blind in one eye, so I need to turn my head pretty far).

It's now been exactly five weeks since my surgery, and I feel almost back to where I was before surgery. I don't tire as quickly, but I've found that my head will start hurting if I do too much straining or walk too "hard."

Andy is another long-time friend in the community who has done more than her share of supporting loved ones through surgeries and illnesses. I was humbled she took the time to write.

ANDY said: You've asked all the right questions and gotten (at least) some of the answers. You're in (otherwise) good health. You've done your medical homework. At this point, the best thing to do is not worry about it. Granted, that is easier said than done, and I don't have a neuroma growing in my head. Live each day with joy, don't sweat the little things, and go on with your day-to-day life the way you ordinarily would. Come February 10, take one day at a time. Worrying over something in the future that, at the moment, you have no control over is a waste of time, energy, and joy, which would be better spent doing what you like. So go do something indulgent instead of getting wound up—it's WAY more fun, anyway!

Barbara is my friend, my walking buddy, and one of our community's spiritual leaders. Her words always inspire me.

BARBARA said: You were created to be human and face the fullness of life. You'll have your difficult moments—that's part of developing compassion. You'll have your drama—it's who you are, no? Take your fears with one hand and your courage with the other, and introduce them to each other. They will show you the way.

Tara is my sister, a nurse. Always practical.

TARA said: 1) Don't worry. 2) Your body will tell you what you can and cannot do after surgery. 3) Get disability as long as you can so you can take some vacations after surgery. 4) Eat a healthy diet. 5) Ask your Dr. to give you pre-op and post-op information.

Marcia is one of a handful of women who I look up to for advice. I hang on every word. This made me cry. I have a hard time believing this is true. Looking different scares me beyond all measure.

MARCIA said: One thought to keep in mind: You will still be you even if you end up looking a little different.

Iris did my hair for a play I was in many years ago. She ratted it up about a foot. When it hurt or I asked her about how to comb it out later, her response became famous.

IRIS said: I volunteer to be your wig person. And remember the famous words, "Don't worry about it."

Do you know people who embody love so well that it oozes out of their pores? This is Gail. Entertaining, comforting, nurturing, supporting, loving, caring, hugging. We met at a wedding and had a connection that cannot be broken. Just thinking about her makes me smile. Always.

GAIL said: Eat? Why, Twinkies, of course! And cookie dough ... and the occasional Oreo milk shake. Silly Woman. Oh ... yeah ... and granola bars. Sheesh ... a tumor shows up, and you forget all the important stuff ... mmmm ... Double Stuff ... THAT'S all the "what" you need.

Ted's not old enough to be my father, but he always gives me fatherly advice. And I appreciate it in just that way.

TED said: You should continue to eat and function the way you do without any changes or breaks in your normal rhythms. Paperwork will take care of itself, thanks to the doctors' staffs. There is no point in worrying or planning for the unknown; that will merely put even more stress on you than you are putting on yourself. You should focus on the fact that you are surrounded by friends and family that love and support you, and know that our collective best wishes are mightier than any other remedy beyond the surgery itself. Is there a support group for people who have already undergone this type of surgery? If not, you might want to create one to share your experience with others, because that's the way you think.

Jeanne and I met through a locally managed teen empowerment program. She is one of the most inspiring, encouraging people I know.

JEANNE said: AHHH!!! NO, NO, NO! And then, YES, YES, YES!

My response: My thoughts exactly.

Susan is a friend who lives across the country. Scrabble is how we stay connected.

SUSAN said: Will you still play a mean game of Scrabble??

MY response: Good question, my friend. That remains to be seen.

Chapter 3. PRESURGERY

December 28, 2009: Bottom 40 countdown

Forty-four days from today I go under the knife. I contemplate the many things I need to do between now and then that I should have done way before this day. Do you have a will? I don't. Do you have a DPOA (Durable Power of Attorney)? I don't. Does your spouse/partner know where all your important stuff is, who the important people in your life are, your passwords to your email, Facebook, computer? And if everything turns out okay, on day forty-five, do you want him or her to have all that information? That is a deeper question, which I will not attempt to answer here. I am just asking.

Besides, we are talking worst-case scenario, right? Everything is supposed to work out just fine. I'm supposed to recover completely after a short mental hiatus, at which time I will re-enter my life, slowly at first, and then at some point in the not too distant future, I'll hopefully be able, and expected, to work and play at the same speed at which I do now.

The question I'm asking myself now is: Do I want to? For the past six months, since my diagnosis, I have made some very carefully thought-out choices as far as what I choose to do and what I choose not to do. Who I choose to spend time with.

How I choose to treat myself and others. It takes time to do that ... time I never had time to do before. I know I'm not dying ... it's not cancer. But there's still that small teeny tiny chance that I will not be the same after and I only have forty-four days to be who I am. Who I am to be. To say what I need to say.

Think about it. If you were told today that in forty-four days your life might be completely different for the rest of your life, what is the first thing you would do? Not to say your life would be worse or better, just different. Your life could change tomorrow and you should live today like it's your last ... fully and with genuine love and appreciation for everyone around you.

Well, that's what I am doing at this very moment. The comments and concerns for my health and well-being are incredibly humbling and overwhelming to me. Every new comment brings me to tears, and I am so grateful.

It occasionally comes up in casual conversation that I am thought of as a strong person. I have lots of shoulders to lean upon. Truly, it is the support and encouragement from my community of friends and family that gives me hope that there will be a day forty-five.

And it will be good.

COMMENTS
Having worked in a probate law firm, I know this comment from Andy is true. Yet here I am without a will. Ridiculous!

ANDY said: I can't stress enough that the will/POA/etc. is not an "if" but a "MUST DO." It's never fun to have to do this kind of thing, but it is essential. Do you really want to leave all that to the whim of the court/medical system? People shouldn't wait until surgery to do this, either. Every adult who has a significant other in their life (be it a spouse, child, partner, sibling, etc.) should have these documents so that their wishes are indeed carried out the way they want them to be. Once that's done, it will be off your "I don't want to deal with this" plate, and you can really relax and enjoy time with everyone.

Jacqui is an old friend from high school. Another friend with her own health issues.

JACQUI said: Each day will bring different questions and different answers even if it's the same question. No matter what answers you come up with, they're the right ones for you because that's what you decided. Do what makes you feel good and puts a smile on your face. That's all that matters.

Adrienne, my friend from Canada, is the voice of experience. I want to be like her someday.

ADRIENNE said: Crazy that it takes these huge life "issues" to remind us of our choices in life and how we choose to spend the rest of our life.

GAIL said: The story doesn't end after the surgery—you're asking really profound questions, and we all want to know the answers.

My response: Why does it take a life threatening illness to ask the hard questions?

Mindy and I have been friends for almost thirty years. She is wise. She has also, suffered her lion's share of health issues and taught me a lot about compassion.

MINDY said: Here is a suggestion: Put a document together with all your passwords, screen names, etc., and put it in an envelope, sealed. Give it to a very trusted friend (you can mail it to me if you want). That way, IF it is needed, it will be available; if it is NOT needed, your trusted friend will destroy the contents. How about that? Also, DO A WILL AND DPOA ... there is not ifs, ands, or butts about it.

More good advice from Ted:

TED said: Wills, DPOAs, trusts if appropriate are all essential tools in this life we lead, regardless of health, but especially because of it. The envelope idea is a good one; if all else fails you can give it to an attorney as a "safe" third party. You could also write out your most intimate thoughts for future sharing in the same manner. Don't forget, spouse, children, parents, etc.— they all have a stake in this and you should be sure you tell them those things you never got around to saying in person. You can always ask for the envelope back and shred it after the surgery is successful … or maybe not.

Dee is one of the many women I look up to in my town. She is a philanthropist, business owner, and all-around kind person. This states the obvious, but still, it speaks to the power I feel in my fear.

DEE said: Conscious choices are really empowering.

———

My mother had experienced breathing difficulty the November after my diagnosis. Her physicians were going back and forth arguing and deciding whether to fix her lung issue through surgery, or first correct her known heart murmur they had found ten years earlier when she had undergone a mastectomy. Each doctor felt the other procedure needed to be done first. I think neither doctor wanted to be responsible for her anticipated surgical complications that were sure to arise as a result of her out-of-control diabetes. Because of all of this, and because she also, just in April of 2009, had undergone a BTK (Below The Knee) amputation of her right foot, she knew she wasn't going to be able to be on my support team and offer any assistance after my surgery. She could barely walk across the room in her own home. How could she possibly walk up the stairs in my house to help take care of me?

January 2, 2010: New Year's Day

This is the year. Forty days from today. I'm enjoying living in the calm before the storm ... not feeling prepared in any way other than having the date of surgery scheduled. Considering how much I have done—exercising, eating right, keeping my personal boundaries—I should feel more prepared than I do.

What I find most interesting is that survivors of this condition/surgery are coming out of the woodwork here in my little hometown. I know of or have already spoken with six survivors here. It's comforting to talk to these people, even though a few have facial nerve damage—it's a future I may have to confront. So I soldier through those conversations and go home and weep. I can't imagine what life is going to be like after my surgery. I know what I want it to be like. I know I'm supposed to imagine the positive, but I'm trying to be realistic and be open to all the possibilities ... good and less than good. Then I weep some more.

Eighteen years ago, when I was pregnant with my son, my mother sat me down and told me that I was "the strong one." That people would always depend upon me and I just had to resign myself to it. I think it took me a long time to come to terms with that and accept and embrace my strength as a duty to my family and my friends. No time or place to be weak or scared or needy. Without reservation or hesitation, I would volunteer, step up, raise my hand, and do my best to help wherever needed. I loved it. I thrived on it. My duty became my drive and my passion.

A surprise response to my online journal is from my mother. She tells me when she reads it, it bothers her that I am scared. That I shouldn't be scared. She doesn't like it when I'm scared. I think it's hard for her to see me scared. I hardly ever seem scared to many people. In person, face-to-face, I deflect, deny, and disregard my fears in exchange for humor. For some reason, it's easier to be honest about being afraid here. Being a mere mortal is going to be a new way of living for me.

I really appreciate the comments that have been left here ...

they are sweet and supportive and make me want to keep sharing what's going on inside my head (literally) with you.

COMMENTS

Stacy is the best friend of my sister Tara.

STACY said: It is time for you, my friend, to lay down your magic wand, cuddle up with your husband and kids, and let the rest just blow away. And it is not only okay, it is healthy and normal that you are scared. You are entitled to be.

Andrea is another friend who lives on the East Coast. Permission to be scared accepted!

ANDREA said: They say true courage is moving ahead even in the face of fear. I'd say it's also knowing when to be scared, and this is one of those times. What makes you strong is your ability to move forward, even in the face of that fear.

Marcia and I have become much closer as a happy outcome of this diagnosis.

MARCIA said: I hear a real identity crisis churning as you anticipate changes in yourself and in your role vis-à-vis family and friends—one our culture does not prepare us for at all—that at some point we start to lose pieces of our looks, our functioning—and how is one supposed to feel about it and cope with the changes? We absolutely ignore this reality in our culture—life is supposed to be a bowl of cherries in America to the end—and of course, it is not, but we are given no tools for dealing with this reality—either as the one going through the changes or as the support cast. I'm just so sorry that you are having to face a crisis of identity so young (over and above the normal sags, etc., everyone has by fifty)—of maybe not being able to maintain your role as the strong, stoic one who can help everyone else through whatever and perhaps having your appearance and some functioning compromised by the surgery itself. It might help (a tiny bit, maybe) to think about how you respond to someone who has a health-related loss; you don't look at them as a lesser person; they are who they are then and there, and you accept them 100 percent just the way they are. Others are much quicker to let go of expectations than the person who actually suffered a loss. How many changes we undergo in self-definition/identity as adults because of the losses along the way and the fact that we really have no/few philosophical frameworks/coping strategies/mantras to latch on to to help us navigate the changes. My wish for you is that whatever happens with this surgery, you will be able to accept the new Marla as is and to comfortably let yourself be freed from some of the layers of expectations you and others have laid on you during your life.

Adrienne, the beacon of hope and experience and success:

ADRIENNE said: Don't over think it. You'll have days where you truly make it through and think "Wow, I thought about it very little today and actually had a really great day—I wasn't pretending!" and other days where you just want to bury your head under a blanket and not come out. It's ALL normal. Just allow yourself to "be." Whatever that may be. There is no manual for this (sucks that there isn't …).

I also think it's smart that even though you're allowing yourself to try to think positive, you also let the "what if's" creep in so that you can picture yourself trying to deal with them.

So many of my friends have had health struggles, it's humbling and a little embarrassing to receive support from people who have their own stuff. Karen, the wife of my husband's college buddy, left words to comfort me, even though I'm not super religious. I'll take all the good wishes I can get.

KAREN said: Rest in the calm that your strength will be there when you need it, and that God allows us to be human in all its foibles. So, allow the fears out. Expect the unexpected. If it all goes according to plan, then you'll be delightfully surprised. Be comfortable not planning out how it will go. Be comfortable knowing only that you are now, and always will be, in the best hands.

My response: So, so true ...

A newer friend, Sherry and I bonded over our love of the word "bitch." As a performer myself, she speaks in language I understand.

SHERRY said: Scared can be your friend. Great artists are scared each time they walk onto the stage. They use their scared friend to be better performers, transforming fear into inspiration.

Jacqui's words also help me understand, in a different way:

JACQUI said: As for your mother, it would be the same for you with your son. I'm sure you would love to protect him so he had no fear either. It's a parent's right to want only good things for your children and take away the bad.

———

January 5, 2010: Preparing to prepare
The strangest thing happened this week. I was at the store, just getting some stuff for a little post-show cast gathering, and I wandered over to the wine section. I was looking for a red, since we had used up all of our wine last month at the Chanukah party. I was not really looking for anything in particular, and then one bottle caught my eye. It was a Cabernet from Australia ... named "Norman's." Yes, that is correct. Of course, I picked up two bottles, one to have, and a second in case it didn't suck. I brought one bottle to my friend Margaret's house party that night, and she and I and a few others shared the bottle. As we toasted a "fond" farewell to Norman, I realized just how

much power there is in goodbye. The time for closure, for ending, for saying and feeling all that is true, leaving nothing out.

And it was good.

And the wine wasn't bad either.

I'm saving the second bottle for after my surgery to drink with my team. We will celebrate and toast Norman off on his trip into oblivion.

Sunday is the thirty-second day before surgery, and I will begin my earnest focus on the surgery itself and becoming physically prepared. I am now walking a few miles at a time about four times a week.

In anticipation of Sunday, I am going to my favorite club and inviting all of my friends to come dance and drink with me. Sunday will be the last day that I will have alcohol, sugar, or wheat until after Norman's eviction.

I always do this sort of thing. A last blowout big meal the day before I start a diet. I might straighten up the house before a new housekeeper (or the regular one) shows up. Or right before I get a haircut, I spend a long time fixing my hair.

I just remember how good I felt over the summer when I had banished all those products from my system ... even though my ear continued to ring. So Saturday will be a celebration evening, in anticipation and preparation of getting my mind and body ready.

Sunday will be the beginning of my getting grounded, to steady my nerves, to find that quiet calm focused energy to sustain me through the next month and the days following surgery.

My friends (what an honor to call them such a thing) Dean and Dudley are producing a workshop on meditational healing, where I will learn how to use musical techniques to reach a deeper state of meditation; how to clear and quiet my mind with sound, breath, toning and positive affirmations for a successful daily meditation practice; and how to create a personal healing mantra and experience chakra toning to balance my energy centers and enhance all aspects of my life.

Of course, this is probably a good idea in general, except I know there are members of my family who will think this is too "woo-woo" and that I have gone over the deep end, will start wearing only tie-dye and grow my hair out into dreadlocks....but hey, I have a brain tumor, so get over it.

COMMMENTS

ANDY said: Don't worry about people thinking that some of your ideas are too "woo woo." You do whatever you want and whatever makes you feel more in control of the situation. Positive mindset goes a LONG way towards the healing process.

My response: Do I need permission? No. Do I appreciate it anyway? You bet. I know, people just want to be helpful. You would not believe (or maybe you would) how many people sent me doctors' names, medical center referrals, medication and diet options, and even websites with all the optional procedures possible for my diagnosis. Interestingly enough, no one sent me the website links for either the U.S. or Canadian Acoustic Neuroma Association, but I already had those.

January 8, 2010: Yes, I did my research and made an informed decision

Consider this the FAQ section. I am sharing why I chose not to opt for some of the following treatment choices. You will not find the intricate specifics of how the many optional acoustic neuroma procedures are done. That's easy enough to find with your best friend, the internet. I'm doing this for two reasons.

First, I want to share all the options that were presented and potentially available to me thanks to hours of searching on the Internet. I searched high and low for information on my condition from "real people" including medical experts and people all over the world who have also had acoustic neuromas to find out what they knew, how they found out, and how they decided what to do.

When I was first looking for information on acoustic neuromas, except for the United States' Acoustic Neuroma Association (ANAUSA) site and the Canada AN sites, there was almost nothing from actual patients except for post-surgical horror stories that I won't go into here. There is no reason to cite "worst case scenarios" for you, my readers. They are easy enough to find and worth skipping here.

Secondly, because I continue to receive suggestions regarding treatment options from friends and acquaintances who, when they hear "acoustic neuroma" and don't know what it is, do what I do and turn to the Internet, I want to thank them, and ask them to stand down.

Believe me, I do my research. Here is a list of the most widely available and used options, and why (or why not) I might have considered them but are not an option for me for addressing my neuroma:

Do nothing. Not an option. My tumor is medium large (2.7cm) and is in a location that is a concern to my doctors. It's very close to my brain stem already, and clearly, to them anyway, wrapped around the nerves. For myself, since my expectation that the symptoms of tinnitus, hearing loss, and balance will only get worse after surgery, I feel I can live with Norman the way he is today. On the other hand, he can change size and shape at any time. Doing nothing was an option only if Norman did not grow or change at all in the six months between the time he was discovered and the second MRI. But he did grow ...

Radiation. Also not an option. Norman is too large and too close to my brain stem. Radiation will make him swell like a marshmallow in the microwave. Just imagining the goo of Norman all over the inside of my head is frightening enough. Even if he were smaller, even if he were not so close to my brain stem, radiation might make his overall consistency harder to remove if I ever did need surgery. No thank you.

Proton. I chose no.

This method is similar to the radiation, but instead of reaching the tumor by going through other healthy brain matter, it circles the tumor so that there is less radiation disturbing innocent parts of the brain. The problem is that no one at the Loma Linda center where they do the proton treatment can confirm or deny whether cystic tumors (like I have) will pop like blisters and spread goo all over my brain.

Endoscopic surgery. I'm not a gambler.

It all sounds very slick at first but then sounds like smoke and mirrors, and I could never find out how much it costs, or which insurance covers it. It's a new kind of approach, done by only one doc in the world, and he's in Los Angeles. Rumor has it he goes in through the nose with a camera-tipped device and extracts the tumor by making a dime-sized hold in your head. Way less invasive than other options. I talked to a few people who wished he had done their surgery, since they lost their hearing. But, I never found or even heard about an actual patient who has had this surgery. There are, however, really cool videos of the surgery on YouTube. (so unless the video is all computer generated, someone must have had this doctor treat them, right?) I have also heard rumors of bad things about the money part of this practice, which makes me nervous. Since I never got a quote of the cost from this practice, all I had heard was that one person almost had this doctor treat him, but after he received a reasonable quote, lots of costs got tacked on when he went in for his pre-op exam. So he never had the surgery. In addition, this doctor has a bad professional reputation among some of his peers. Even though all of that may just be gossip, I decided to not talk to him.

Sub fossa. Not an option.

Norman is just too large for this surgery.

I have narrowed it down to two choices:

Translaborynthe: This is the treatment most of the doctors recommended for me. It is apparently the "easiest" in that it usually takes less time, and it is easier for the surgeons to see what they are doing around the nerves. There is not any possibility to preserve any hearing on the side of the surgery. The post-surgical complications are about the same for this one and the retrosigmoid (see below). And the packing—the bandage—for the after surgery is HUGE! It sticks out about three inches from the ear and wraps around the top of the head and the chin like a mummy.

Middle fossa—retrosigmoid: Only Dr. Superman recommends this course of action for me, and it seems to be his preferred method of surgery, as the other two of his patients I met had the same procedure. The other doctors I met say that this is not their preferred option because of the potential for post-surgical headaches. They also don't guarantee they can save any of my hearing anyway, so it's not worth the risk. Dr. Superman thinks he might be able to save some hearing, and it's worth the chance. I might end up having headaches, which does not thrill me, but given a choice between not ever hearing music or birds or whispers in my left ear for the rest of my life, I am okay with the gamble on this one. If I lose my hearing anyway, at least I can say I tried, right?

And because I may permanently lose the hearing in my left ear after the surgery, I am planning, preparing, proactively doing SOMETHING ... I plan to store up whispers in my left ear. So I ask everyone I know to whisper something in my left ear that I will be able to hold in my heart and memory if and when I can no longer hear in that ear.

Okay, so there you have it.

COMMENTS

ADAM said: I like the "marshmallow in the microwave" analogy —that's also one of the reasons I opted against radiation for now. I may revisit radiation once mine has been de-bulked, but it's also too big right now. I also decided endoscopic was not the way to go—that doc in L.A. is too "Hollywood" for me, and he's not a board-certified neurosurgeon. The small incision and small hole sounds appealing, however, that becomes a real liability if the patient starts bleeding heavily. Supposedly it can be near impossible to stop bleeding in some situations without doing a craniotomy—if you already have a craniotomy, you're way ahead of the game, right? Thank you for sharing your rationale. It's neat to hear another patient making the same decisions.

My response: I didn't think I need to be validated, but after these comments, I actually felt better!

Heidi is one of those "earth-mama" types who never seems to get ruffled when faced with a challenge. I know this isn't true, which makes her all that much stronger in my eyes.

HEIDI said: You sort of have to earn your own med. degree in an effort to make the best decision. I'm glad you have the resources to do this research!

My response: Truly, I feel like I have learned a lot, and it helps me believe I have made the right decision. For me. I am lucky to have had the time and resources to do this research.

Marian is my scientific, practical, engineering friend.

MARIAN said: Solid descriptions, Marla—not the least boring for me—your review of options is just the way this project engineer would go about it.

January 9, 2010: Woo-woo weekend

I attend the meditational healing workshop that my friends put on. It is pretty full… about thirty people in attendance. I think two of us are not experienced at meditating, but the leaders are kind enough to baby step us into "how to" while everyone there participates. For the first guided meditation, we inhale for four counts, hold for eight, then exhale for eight. At one point, the leader says something during the guided meditation. I can't even remember exactly what she said, but I get a full head and body rush and start tearing up. I breathe. I calm down. When we open our eyes, she is looking at me and is smiling. She knows. Sigh. The rest of the whole two-hour workshop is like this. We take a break. The store we are doing the workshop in has lots of books, stones, smudging sticks (for clearing bad vibes out of a living or working space), and stuff like that. Break is over and the group is brought back together. We are then guided to do something called chakra focusing, which I have never even heard of, much less experienced before. Chakras correspond to vital points in the physical body such as organs, arteries, veins, and nerves. (I guess I'm not as "woo woo" as I thought—the fact that I didn't know this already is very telling.) Okay, stay with me here. We chant by focusing on color and sound for each of the seven chakras, starting at the base of the spine and moving all the way to the top of the skull. I don't get what the first three even mean, but once I get to the heart chakra, I feel like I am able to get a bit of a grasp on each one that follows. I'm not sure if what I feel was right, but it is something, and so I just assume I am doing okay. I have no idea if it means my chakras are "open"—or what even that means—but I ask the leaders and am assured I am normal. As if.

At the end of the workshop, we practice mantras (power statements). Most of them are in other languages, and we chant them a little bit. Then Dudley shares one she wrote for herself (in English) when she was suffering from dizziness and ear ringing. No, she did not have a tumor; hers went away like normal people's do, but thank you for asking. When she repeats her mantra, she looks at me, and my insides go weak. It is perfect. Its power is tangible. Um, no, I can't remember her mantra, but ...

At the very end, she goes around the circle and asks us to give our feedback of the workshop in one word, and the group will repeat the word to reinforce it. I am almost near the end of the circle, so I really have time to think about it. The first word that pops into my head is "ready," as in "ready for surgery," which is so typical of me to jump in feet first ... I am so not ready, but I'm working on it, right? So then I re-think and come up with "focused," as in, I'm planning, preparing, and getting ready, right? So I've got my word, I'm all excited because lots of people are saying the same types of things—grateful, peaceful, calm—they get to me ... and I cannot remember my word. Oy. What's worse: I finally do remember, and the word is "focused" Well, I am lost for words.

I will carve out some time for myself this week to practice my new hobby of meditation. And it will be good.

COMMENTS

GAIL said: So ... I did that "in for four, hold for eight, out for eight" breath thingy? Got dizzy ... good that I was already sitting down ... Sheesh ... Kick Norman's ass to the curb. Still dizzy ...

My response: See, isn't she funny?

———

January 11, 2010: Thirty days and counting

Today is the tenth. In thirty days, on February 10, I will show my faith and trust in the physicians and nurses and prayers and supporters and caregivers and just let go and let them do their jobs.

When I woke up this morning and looked at the calendar, my stomach dropped a little bit. My head spun, and I sat very still and tried to breathe normally.

Could have been because the night before we had the formal going away party for Norman. Not a formal in the sense of tuxedos and long dresses. This was a kickoff party to start the organized planning and making of arrangements to ensure that Norman's demise and my recovery from it will be safe and sane and forever. This was a party!

One of my favorite dance bands was playing at a local dance club, and I invited everyone I knew to come dance him a fond farewell with me. Oh, by the way, in preparation for surgery, since I've decided I won't be drinking any alcohol for the next thirty days either, some of my friends took this to mean that they wanted/needed to buy me a last glass of wine for a while. I had six of them. Oy. Yeah, Norman hated me this morning...

Feeling mortal, I realized that I'd really better get on that bucket list of life experiences. A little backstory here: I'd lived in my little town for well over fifteen years and had had fleeting moments of fame at the local television station. Which, over the fifteen years I knew of it, and the fifteen-plus years before that, had seen a steady decline in local programming. One self-produced weekly show remained at KVOS, which is now, sadly, no longer local. At that time, "Experience Northwest with Deb Slater" had a following, a YouTube channel, and a Facebook page. Early in January, Deb and I were chatting on Facebook, going back and forth about a few things, and she asked me about the date of that workshop I was planning to attend. I made some snarky comment to her about reading my journal more carefully, and she shot back a comment that made me realize I had hurt her feelings. I felt sick to my core. I mean, why would I think she was supposed to have my schedule committed to memory? Even I didn't. So I quickly pulled myself together, drove to the market, picked up some fresh flowers, and went to her studio. When she saw me with the flowers, she smiled and brought me upstairs to her office.
She showed me her show board—work board, or whatever it's called—and said, "Look at my board. Look at it."
I looked at it, and it was very white. It had some nice white space. I nodded yes.
She said, "You don't know what it means, do you?"
I said, "No." Heck, I didn't even know what it was.

41

She said, obviously distressed, "It means I have ten minutes to fill for the show this weekend, and I don't know what I'm going to do."

Jumping at the chance to help a friend in need, I said, "I can help you. I'll fill a minute." I did not know what this meant or what it would entail.

"What do you mean?"

I quickly made up something and said, "I'll talk about something for a minute."

"What are you going to talk about?"

I said (honestly), "I don't know. I'll think of something"

She looked at me for a quick minute and said, "For one minute?"

"Yes"

Then she thought about it ... for less than a minute ...and she said, "What are you going to call it?"

"GimmeAMinute."

She said okay.

And that's how "GimmeAMinute" started.

January 13, 2010: Day twenty-eight

It's been a good day, a hard day, and a great day. Even though today was the day I found out that my sister, who is a nurse, could not stay with me after my surgery for as long as I thought. I was counting on her to be my caretaker, my control freak, my mother-knows-best Nurse Ratched until I was completely recovered. (And that was all in my head—she never said she could or would do that ... stupid Norman.) My surgery is on a Thursday. She's leaving the following Tuesday. I don't even know if I'll be home by then! I had somewhat of a meltdown, and then this morning I realized I really have amassed a great team of women friends to help me after I come home. I trust them to know what to do, who to call, if they or I need help beyond what they are or I am capable of. I let that stress go first thing this morning, and it totally revitalized my day.

Then, this afternoon, I had lunch with my friend Adrienne, one of the two women I met online through the AN forum and in person at the Canadian symposium. Since we met face-to-face in September, she's been following my journey through my journal and has occasionally left great supportive comments and has given me powerful feedback. We have talked at length about the days following her surgery, her support team, her post-surgery issues. It was comforting and informational. I have a better idea of what to expect, best-case scenario. Plus, it helps so much to know that there are positive outcomes to the surgery. Her surgery was four months after she found out about her tumor.

After spending that hour with her today, I have increased hope. Meanwhile, my bucket list continues to get shorter. My first GimmeAMinute is being broadcast locally as a fill piece on my friend Deb Slater's show. I am like a TV correspondent, like Andy Rooney, Jane Curtin, Gilda Radner, Amy Poehler … okay, maybe I'm only a wannabe, but it is fun and exciting, and it's soon to be available online! The first GimmeAMinute will be posted on the Internet on January 18.

Thinking about the possibility of not being able do that, to write and produce another GimmeAMinute again is sad. If my thought process doesn't work, if my face doesn't work…it's the most frightening prospect of everything. After we had recorded the six segments that first day in the studio, Deb looked at the calendar and pointed to a date six weeks after my surgery is scheduled, and she wrote me in on the studio schedule for that day.

I have to admit, while it felt good, comforting, and hopeful to make plans for "after," I am still uneasy.

But Deb is sweet and is keeping it positive and is completely confident.

So I let myself live in that moment … a little.

We'll see Ms. Slater … You'll have to speak to my agent.

COMMENTS

Molly is another woman I met when our kids went to school together. She's smart and funny and very direct. Like me, which is why being the third wheel around us can be a little intimidating. She helped me name this book.

MOLLY said: As I read your stress concerning your post op, I couldn't help but remember back to the early seventies and "sensitivity training," where we would allow ourselves to fall into the waiting arms of our friends. We are here, and we WILL lift you up!

I adore this woman ... this comment cracked me up:

DEB said: Agent? Good lord. I've created a monster.

———

January 17, 2010: Twenty-five days and counting ... quickly

I know I talk quickly ... I am constantly asked to repeat myself or slow down when I speak; however, I don't think I speak half as fast as the time is passing. Just so you know, in my head it doesn't seem like I'm speaking half as fast as I actually am. I think that's why I am always speeding up. There is so much to say, so much to do, before I can take a break from everything.

As I get closer to surgery, I'm noticing more aches in my head. Is the tumor growing faster now too? Am I just acutely aware of Norman's existence? Is he ready to leave and trying to work his way out of my ear all by himself? And my head is starting to feel spinny more often, as if I've had a rush of adrenaline. Is it really my blood pressure this time? Is it Norman eating more of the vestibular nerve? If my balance nerve is totally gone by February 10, and I have compensated for it all this time, will I be able to walk without assistance that first day after? According to my sister, the nurse who knows everything, I will be fine and dandy after surgery. I am a bit less sure, although I'm still planning for a less than desired outcome "just in case," so that my psyche will be able to relax.

Over the past few weeks, I have been seeing friends, getting nice get-well-don't-worry cards and calls, going out for walks, out to lunch, tea, music, dancing, etc. I am busier than ever and running out of time. I'm burning the candle at both ends, which might explain why I have a sore throat and a runny nose.

I met with another local woman who is a surgery survivor this week. She had the same surgery I did, but over ten years ago. A short time after her first symptom, she was diagnosed and had her surgery within three months. She had many post-surgical issues, not least of which was steroid psychosis, where she felt and thought she saw things that weren't really there. Yeah, that sounds like a trip and a half. I'm hoping they have the steroid issues figured out better after my surgery, that's all I can say. She also had the misfortune of having her tumor grow back, so she underwent radiation for the second procedure.

She did lose all the hearing in her left ear and has some facial numbness, but no muscle weakness. And she is a musician! She kept encouraging me to "live my life" and "go on with" my life and just "move on as if nothing happened" after the surgery.

While I appreciate being able to talk with survivors who have had little or no permanent disabling or disfiguring results, I learn as much, if not more, from the folks who have had nerve damage, facial weakness, and persistent and disabling dizziness who still consider themselves AN sufferers. It helps me to meet all these post-surgical survivors, and I look forward to joining their ranks soon.

The fact that I have taken so much time to research my options has left me with the anxiety that maybe I waited too long. It seems like most of the people who have symptoms so severe that they seek treatment and choose to have their surgery well within six months of diagnosis. That is, those from the United States. I guess I won't know if I waited too long until the eleventh, if ever.

COMMENTS

Cheryl is the other woman from Canada I met back in the fall. This advice sat with me for a few weeks but was very helpful.

CHERYL said: I know it is extremely scary facing surgery, and no one ever tells you what you can do while you wait. If I can suggest one option, try to imagine yourself in top shape after the surgery doing something you love. As many times a day as you can and especially right before bed and as soon as you wake up. Really imagine the feeling of everything being good, face intact, smiling, hugging your friends, etc. When we focus on the symptoms, the symptoms will intensify. I know it seems next to impossible at this point, but if you can put yourself in a relaxed state and imagine only the best health and recovery for yourself and really allow yourself to feel it, this will help.

———

January 24, 2010. Three weeks, 21 days, 504 hours, 30, 240 minutes, 1, 814, 400 seconds

That's a lot of seconds. I can get lots done between now and then.

Friday is my last day of work pre-surgery. I decided to give myself two weeks to get things done around the house—paperwork, pre-op stuff, getting the house ready for me and the caregivers by cleaning and moving chairs and clothes and things. I'm also flying to L.A. this weekend to see old friends and my family ... still working on that bucket list. I know my office mates are going to suffer a hardship at the beginning when I am gone, but I also know that no one is indispensable, and they will learn to live without me for a short while. They will also probably find any screwups I have done in the past six months (do you think I might have been a bit distracted?), and maybe they won't even want me to come back. It all remains to be seen. For now, I am working on letting go.

I'm making this trip to Southern California so I can visit with my mom and my sister and brother and their families. I'm going to a big fancy-schmancy birthday dinner with old friends from junior high school, and I'll also hopefully connect with some dear old friends who moved to L.A. from Bellingham. When I come back, it's going to be a quick snowball ride to surgery, the kind that starts off slowly with pre-ops, blood work, stress tests, and all the other things they have to do to determine if I can survive the surgery before they even get to remove Norman and then accelerates to the speed of sound as it reaches check-in at the hospital on the day of the surgery.

I spent part of this morning reflecting on the timing of Norman's first appearance and how many years it took for a diagnosis. I have been adjusting to living with him, as much as I try to adjust to the expectations of living without him, whether the outcome is good or bad. I continue to learn much about myself and my ability and need to ask for help and support, and have realized how powerful and humbling it has been to be able to do that—both for myself, and for the people I feel "safe" to ask.

Meanwhile, under the category of "what did you do today to prepare for surgery," my friend Anji sent me this poem. It's by Rumi. I think it's in place of the whisper, but I'll take it. I wanted to share it.

Bird Wings

Your grief for what you've lost lifts a mirror
up to where you're bravely working.
Expecting the worst, you look,
and instead, here's the joyful face you've been wanting
to see.
Your hand opens and closes and opens and closes,
If it were always a fist or always stretched open,
you would be paralyzed.
Your deepest presence
is in every small contracting and expanding,
the two as beautifully balance and coordinated
as bird wings.

COMMENTS
Of course Ted is worried about his buddy part of our couple friendship:

TED said: We are thinking positive thoughts for Ken; it's never easy to watch a loved one go through a personal crisis, but it's also possible to become invisible when everyone is focusing on the person with the problem.

BARBARA said: This is all part of the opening and closing that the poem refers to. Here's another for you, from Rilke's Book of *Hours: Love Poems to God* by Rainer Maria Rilke (translators: Barrows and Macy)

> God speaks to each of us as he makes us, then walks
> with us silently out of the night.
> These are the words we dimly hear:
> You, sent out beyond your recall, Go to the limits of
> your longing. Embody me.
>
> Flare up like flame and make big shadows I can move
> in. Let everything happen to you: beauty and terror. Just
> keep going. No feeling is final. Don't let yourself lose me.
> Nearby is the country they call life. You will know it
> by its seriousness.
> Give me your hand.

January 22, 2010: I am very lucky ...
I know that. I only have an acoustic neuroma. It has made me aware of what else I have, and how things could be way, way worse.

I don't have cancer.

I don't live in Haiti.

I have a roof over my head, food in the refrigerator, and enough money in the bank to pay my bills.

I have medical insurance.

I have an excellent team of doctors taking the absolute best care of me.

I am married to a good man.

I have great kids.

I have a fantastic family.

I have unbelievable friends who care about me and will help me when I need it.

Yes, call me lucky. And very grateful. And humbled ...

COMMENTS

Todd is married to Anji, who also posts very introspective poetry. I have read these lines over and over and have seen and felt something different each time. I've never really been a huge aficionado of this kind of writing, but lately it seems to fit in my life.

TODD said: True courage is the product of tenderness. It arises when we let the world touch our heart, Our heart that is so beautiful and so bare. We are ready to open ourselves up, with no resistance or timidity, And truly face the world. We are ready to share our heart with others. (Chogyam Trungpa)

And then, of course, I get these lines by my dear friend who knows my love of theater and movies and musicals.

SYLVIA said: I never tire of Bing and Rosemary singing, "If you're worried and you can't sleep, then count your blessings instead of sheep," over a pitcher of buttermilk ...

January 27, 2010: Two weeks

I usually sleep on the couch in the family room when I visit my family in California in the San Fernando Valley. But I am writing this from my niece's bedroom. She has given up her bedroom for me, and she's sharing a bunk bed with her little brother, my nephew, just so I can sleep in a room with a door that closes. This allows me to wake up without her dog sticking her nose in my face. Everyone is making such sacrifices for me these days ...

49

Over the past few days, I was able to fit in some quality time with a small group of old friends that I've known since way back in junior high!! I walked by my old house, the one I grew up in, which my mom sold a few years ago. All the flowers we planted in the front of the house that I loved are gone ... no more gardenias, star jasmine, roses, climbing vines by the garage. They have been replaced with palm trees and succulents. As much as I don't like what they have done, it's clearly not my house anymore, so it's easer to let go. Closure.

I attempt to get a whisper in my ear out of my mom. My sister whispers, "I will always be younger than you," "You are beautiful, I am younger." We find the humor wherever we can. My mother cannot quite get the hang of whispering. She just talks to me in a normal-volume voice. She never could whisper. Once in a not-very-full movie theater, she and I were watching a film, and she turned to me and said, "This is boring." Everyone in the room heard her. We left. Once, while waiting for an event at my daughter's elementary school to begin, another child was playing the piano as people were finding their seats. She turned to me and said, "He's awful." His parents were sitting in front of us. They still give me the stink-eye when they see me.

Even now, when given specific instructions by my sister, my mother still cannot whisper in my ear. It is a memory in itself ...

I woke up in a panic in the middle of the night. What if I picked the wrong doctors? What if the neurosurgeon sneezes during my surgery? What if there is an earthquake during my operation? What if?

I'm not sure if the "what ifs" came before I woke up or after. But it took me a little while to get back to sleep. Yeah, I still get scared sometimes, but I think back to how I felt in June, July, and August. I remember how many times I would find myself having what I referred to as "a moment," where I became so utterly terrified that I didn't know what to do next. It paralyzes me.

Then, I started distracting myself with living. And it has been an amazing thing, to really savor every moment with friends, with family, with myself. One of the things the neurosurgeon said to do to get myself as physically ready as possible was to increase my cardio activity. I'm sure he thinks I will be doing aerobics, biking, or running, but I have been so lethargic for the past year, I just do a lot of walking. I am blessed with friends who are willing to walk with me. Nancy, Mish, Francie (who can outrun the Roadrunner on a good day), Susan, Elizabeth, Jo, Barbara ... all of these women join me in early morning walks and talks, which help me, support me, encourage me, and are such gifts to me for the past few months. I am eternally grateful for this time we spend together.

Just before I came on this trip, I walked by myself because I was too lazy to call someone to walk with me. Well, actually, that's not true. I have been working up to walking alone for years. This time, I walked around Lake Padden, a well-traveled and loved running trail. I walked clockwise, the opposite way most people walk and run the lake. I figured I'd maximize the possibility that I would cross paths with another human. And I did, and yet I felt totally safe in an environment of solitude. Later on that day, I took another leisurely walk on the waterfront. I was in heaven. Lots of time for introspection—not that the conversation with my walking partners hasn't been introspective as well, but I finally was able to have a conversation with myself, to really acknowledge how far I have come in the past six months, both physically and emotionally. I even chanted my mantra a little bit!

I know the next fourteen days are going to fly by. Every day is filling up with people to see, things to do, whispers to receive. Keep them coming. I am so grateful for them.

COMMENTS

Lauralee reached out to me shortly after my diagnosis. Her son had gone through something similar (but not the same), and she was very comforting. I'm grateful to surgeons' moms too!

LAURALEE said: I am grateful to those surgeons' moms who supported them through med school and am praying for their steady hands and best judgments.

One of the things I took away from the local small group acoustic neuroma meetings was the need to get ahead of the vestibular (balance) therapy. Ann, my primary care doctor who I love and appreciate more every day for her support and willingness to truly partner with me in my medical care, gave me a referral for a physical therapist for vestibular assessment and exercises. They checked my current level of balance (and imbalance) and gave me exercises to do prior to and immediately after surgery.

January 31, 2010: A perfect ten

I have ten days to go. My bucket lists are basically done! I have one sewing project to complete; bills to pay; furniture to rearrange; last-minute walks, lunches, and doctor's appointments to attend; balance exercises and blogging to do, shopping lists to make for my husband, one cash card to acquire for my son, and plane reservations to make for the two of them to go to San Francisco to see the play my daughter is directing in March. I'll get a ticket for myself too, but I'm buying insurance on that ticket, just in case.

I don't know why I end up writing and posting in the middle of the night. During the day, I think about things that I want to share, and then it gets to be 11:00 PM, midnight, 1:00 AM, and I realize the day is gone and if I don't do this now, I may lose a whole other day and then forget what I wanted to say.

Friday morning I was gifted a massage by Beth, who is a new friend since the summer. Not only is Beth a great masseuse, she also works on visualization. It seems everyone who crosses my path these days does! We imagined Norman drying up, shrinking in size, going from the size of a walnut to the size of an almond, being so lacking of moisture and adhesiveness that when the surgeon goes in to extract him, he literally pops out of my head!! Okay, maybe the description was a little more graphic, but I don't want to offend anyone or gross them out, so I'll just leave it at that!

Saturday, I met with Dudley, my friend who ran the meditational healing workshop I took a few weeks ago. She had agreed to meet with me privately and do a one-on-one session to help me develop my personal mantra and chant to help sustain me through this process of pre and post surgery. I must say I had no idea how much emotional toll this would take on me.

I have always believed that illness is a manifestation of emotional trauma. I don't believe you can wish or pray things away, though I know there are people out there who do. It's just not what I believe. For me, the identification of the initial symptoms and their connection to what was going on in my life at that time helps me establish "where these things come from." Here is my personal awareness moment, my "aha!" if you will. I told Dudley about two jobs I had accepted in my life that I actively did not love—jobs I took because I felt it was what I was supposed to do. Once in Southern California, and once in Bellingham, I accepted employment at businesses where I knew immediately I did not fit, and both times, I was fired. Both were blows to my ego to be sure, even though I breathed a sigh of relief that I didn't have to work at either place anymore. The karma was bad at each place, and I was so much happier to not be working there. What I remembered/realized today was that the first ear pain came when I left that job in Southern California, and the hearing loss and return of the ear pain returned at the end of the job in Bellingham. Ear pain, loss of hearing, dizziness ... all that, both times. Strange. Odd. Coincidence?

Dudley and I were discussing my current symptoms and how they related to changes in my physical and emotional environment, and the strangest thing happened. The ringing intensified! I told Dudley that around the time Norman made himself known to me this most recent time, in the fall of 2008, I had just begun a period of self-awareness and self-care to a degree I never had my whole life. I had spent a focused two weeks where I got regular exercise, ate right, and was generally happy. Then the intense ringing and hearing distortion started. Since then, I have become even more committed to taking better care of myself, both physically and emotionally, and I have Norman's appearance and soon-to-be exit to thank for that.

Normally in the face of too much conflict and resistance, I would either bolt or go back to the way things were and just hope they miraculously resolved themselves. I know this is not the way I need to deal with Norman.

So what did I learn today? How am I different in this moment than I was when I woke up? How is my life changed from my new knowledge? I don't know that I can answer that in a way anyone can understand completely, but I do know this: There is something, that I am, and that it is.

COMMENTS

ANN said: Again, I am always humbled by my patients knowing more about support systems than I do. So here is another wish for precision in excision and a light-speed recovery.

My response: Precision in excision. Love this!

MARCIA said: Hold onto those thoughts about the positive changes Norman has been/might be a catalyst for.

My response: From bad there always is good. You just have to look deeper.

Pat was my college roommate who has faced more challenges and always returns better and stronger.

PAT said: Remember life keeps the challenges coming so when all the good stuff comes our way we don't take it for granted.

I asked Mish to help me take care of my family while I was out of commission by organizing meals for us for a few weeks. I've participated in preparing meals for other families. It was hard for me to ask, but I have two boys at home, a guy's gotta eat, and I couldn't fathom that much take-out Chinese food or pizza, which is what we would have ended up with until I was back in the kitchen.

Also, because I might need help getting around the house while Ken and Caleb are at work and in school, I might need to have people stop by and hang out if I need something. Sort of like adult babysitting. But just in case.

So seven days before my surgery, I give Mish the password to my online blog so she can keep my friends updated while I'm in recovery. She has set up an online schedule to coordinate my after-surgery care and meals. We called the helpers the FUN crew, for "F--- Y-- Norman." The schedule filled up FAST. I am humbled and overwhelmed. I will never be able to pay everyone back for this, and it makes me sad. Which makes some of my friends a little annoyed. I mean, let's say things were in reverse and a friend or a friend of a friend of mine needed me. Would I expect payback? No! So there!

All we can do is keep breathing.

February 2, 2010: Marla's F.U.N. Food Crew

Hi All: This is Mish, not Marla. I'm sneaking in behind Marla's back to ask those of you in Whatcom County for a favor:

Many of you have voiced an interest in helping Marla out during her recovery. Here's something you can do! Express your love with food, in the grand Jewish tradition! We are looking for people who would like to prepare a meal or two (think dinner) and bring it over to the Bronstein's to take the load off of Ken and Caleb and to help put Marla's mind at ease.

Some food preferences: No Brussels sprouts, no cilantro, no lima beans, no spaghetti. Ken needs to know if any of the dishes have a lot of cheese or milk in them. It's fine if they do, he just needs to take a Lactose pill first. Marla is hoping for fruits and veggies, too. The gal is going to need her vitamins! Keep in mind: Caleb is not picky, but the boy can eat. Also, don't forget cooking instructions, as applicable.

Thanks for doing this. F. U. Norman! —Mish

... now back to your regularly scheduled programming.

DREW said: No Brussels sprouts! You guys are missing the best things in our garden right now!

My response: She started it ...

JILL said: Dang, I have the best recipe for Brussels with cilantro sauce garnished with lima beans. I guess I'll have to save that one when you come over for dinner, Mish!

My response: ... and she kept it going. BTW. I hate cilantro. My friends (and strangers sometimes) give me crap about it. I. DON'T. CARE.

KEN said: Jill, that recipe sounds GREAT to me!!

MARLA said: *(this is the only comment I left after my post in this journal—I hate these vegetables that much)* Jill, that is disgusting.

———

February 3, 2010, 12:29 AM: Overwhelmed
MISH again: You people are too much. I am seriously stunned by how fast Marla's food sign-up filled up.

To everyone who signed up: thank you, thank you, thank you!

We're all hoping that Marla will be up to speed by the time mid-March rolls around. If not, don't worry—I'll let you know.

Marla has such a big warm blanket of love from all of you—

I'm so touched. Keep it up—your good thoughts and words make such a difference to her.

Eight days …

Shirley is my mom. This doesn't really fit here, or maybe it does. Anyway, it was her first time posting, and I just wanted to prove that she's really reading this. So I left it.

COMMENTS

SHIRLEY said: I love you. Was finally able to use this so I am sending you this message. I love you. Mom.

My response: I love you too.

February 3, 2010: All we can do is keep breathing

Let me start by echoing Mish. I am completely overwhelmed with the support and love you have all shown me. Those of you who are taking time out of your lives to care for me, to feed my family, your gifts are greatly appreciated and I don't know how I can ever repay you. Your comments on these pages lift my sprits and give me encouragement to keep sharing with you. Thank you for humoring me and my need to process. You have no idea how much it means to me.

Today has been a strange day. I've crossed many things off my list of things to do. I spent some quality time with a dear friend on her birthday, forged out a new walk path, spent time in one of my favorite parks watching the sun set over the sound, and signed my will, finally! I should have been ecstatic. But then, today had its stresses as well. Another dear friend underwent major surgery to deal with stage 3b uterine cancer. The doctors think they got it all, which is the great news. Two other friends continue their battles with ovarian cancer, but they are fighters as well, and they are determined to beat it. So overall, today was emotionally intense.

What is strange is that I've been in a kind of underlying, deep seated, "I really would rather spend some time by myself" funk all day. I decided to use the moment and examine why I felt that way. Here's what I came up with: The "funk" is the way I deal with stress, my regular habit of responding to something intense. I have been reflective, introspective, in a self-absorbed and generally antisocial way—so different from how I have been for the past few months. I mean, I have been reflective and introspective, but haven't I shared *all of that* with all of you? I mean, at this point, what secrets do I really have?

I spent time alone at a park this afternoon. I turned down an opportunity to go out tonight. I seriously considered not spending time with friends later this week. But I don't want to start down that spiral. I mean, it's okay to take a night off. I'll give myself permission, but, and this is the hard part for me, I will accept the graces of precious time offered to me by my friends. I will be grateful for the time spent on walks, drinking tea, talking, and just being with people.

The more I thought about the timing of this funk, the more clear the reason for it became: Until I scheduled my surgery, I never had a specific date in mind when it would take place. So I had been ruminating on dates as early as January all the way through the summer. When I met my surgeon in December, the tentative date of the surgery was first scheduled for February 3. Within four days, the surgery date was changed because he was going to be out of town. By that time, I had given my notice at work and made plans to go to L.A. I guess I have been carrying that original date around in my head and heart.

I felt like I have been freaking out all day! Not hysterically, not like I was going to faint from fear, but my subconscious never got the memo that the original date had been changed. So once I acknowledged what was happening and why, I started my controlled relaxation breathing, I became calm, and then I was exhausted from all the wasted energy. Damn internal clock!

So all that being said, and being in a better, more social place as

I close down for the evening, one other thing has surfaced today. I will illustrate this with a personal request:

If you know anyone else in Bellingham or in your circle of friends who has had treatment for acoustic neuroma and you have not already connected us through email or phone, I am going to ask you to wait to do that until after my surgery. I have just been connected to survivor #11 in Bellingham. She and I will meet on Thursday, and I already have a feeling her post-surgical results were not stellar. Let me tell you, horror stories are not helping. Not even when this person says, "Oh, don't worry, this will *not* happen to you."

I mean truly, how does one person think sharing their horror stories will support me? I know, knowing all the facts and possibilities should help me prepare for every eventuality. Approach every game as if your life depended on it, and play to win. Well, I am playing to win too. And I ask that you keep your negative comments and stories to yourself. This is a really important part of my visualization and positive thinking approach. I don't need to hear anymore about what negatives are possible. I know many of them already, and I choose to anticipate the better possibilities. I apologize if this sounds harsh, but truly, this is a common circumstance that occurs when people face a medical crisis. Thank you for your understanding.

COMMENTS

And then my friends gave me "permission" to cancel this date:

BARBARA said: Yup—I totally get what you're saying about the horror stories. I think sometimes people don't know what to say, or they think they're coming alongside of you and know what you're going through. For some, until they live it, they don't get it. Good for you for asking for what you need. And as for the meeting with this person on Thursday—you could cancel it. You could talk to her after the surgery or not at all. You call the shots.

I only know Lily as we are both subscribers and commenters to an on-line podcast and have shared music as a result of that. And yet, I was thrilled and flattered she felt so compelled to reach out to me directly this way.

LILY said: There's nothing wrong with wanting to spend some alone or me time right now. People, even the best, most loving, most well-meaning people, can sometimes be a bit much, especially when they're all concerned. So take some time. Those people will still be there when you come back.

And as for horror stories—it's like childbirth. Women will tell you all kinds of stuff that they went through to "prepare" you. Shut up!

Sweet Anne, has survived Hitler's Germany and cancer, and yet always has a smile on her face and time for friends. I adore and honor and am in awe of this woman. An excellent example for setting boundaries!

ANNE said: You don't have to meet with this person tomorrow. This is the time to just do what's best for you!

My father-in-law's girlfriend. She has always been very positive.

CHARLOTTE said: Think your inner wisdom is right-on. No need to hear anything negative when you're working so hard to stay "on the other side"!!

ANDY said: Marla: I'm with you on the visualization! Eye on the prize, babe—eye on the prize!

HEIDI said: Your last paragraph makes me think of women who tell their horrific labor stories to a woman about to give birth for the first time. What are they thinking? I'm so glad you have the presence of a survival mind to block those stories!

JACQUI said: No horror stories from this side of the world. Speaking from a medical perspective, remember you are strong and visualize a positive outcome. That will help carry you through. Amazing how much that really does help. Also know that the support from your family, friends, and family friends will always be there to help you float when you think you're sinking. Positive thoughts coming your way. Show Norman he's a goner!

February 6, 2010: Oh my! I forgot to sleep

Let's file this under the "things I forgot to do when I was burning at both ends" category, shall we? I am four days out from surgery day, and somehow, the universe guided me to keep this day completely open, except for a meeting with Dudley. Since four is my number, I suppose that's no accident. Today could not have come at a better time.

I am exhausted. Emotionally. Physically. I looked at my schedule for the next four days and realized I have no walks on the calendar. Then I realized the only way I can fit them in is if I start at seven in the morning. We'll see if I can drag myself out of bed that early, especially when I don't sleep in the middle of the night. Other than that, I have nothing solid on the calendar. Nothing I have to do. Oh, you know, little chores here and there, but a sweet, easy day. In anticipation of the next three days, I think I will take advantage of my situation (I have a tumor, have you heard?) and delegate everything I can. Oh, let me correct that. There is one other thing on the agenda for today: a nap.

Thursday's meeting with #11 went off almost exactly as I had feared. When she first got out of her car and our eyes met, we smiled in acknowledgment. Well, she half smiled. My stomach dropped. I wanted to run back into my car, but our mutual friend had said she was a lovely person, so I didn't. We introduced ourselves and went into the coffee shop, I got my tea, and we sat down and started talking. Well, to be perfectly correct, she started talking. She asked me how I found out I had a tumor.

After I gave her the Reader's Digest version, she didn't ask me what else I wanted her to know, she didn't ask me if I had any questions about her journey, or her outcomes, or anything.

She just started to tell me.

About her diagnosis, her tumor growth, the size on surgery, the cutting of the facial nerve, the physical therapy, her future that contains seemingly endless surgeries. There appeared to be no possibly favorable outcome to her hopelessness, pain, or frustration. I stopped her and said, "Are you trying to scare me?" This almost, but not quite, stopped her. At that point, my head was spinny, and I just needed to get away.

I had the good foresight to contact two friends earlier in the day and set up an "escape call" about thirty minutes into my scheduled meeting. They agreed to call me. I could choose to ignore the call, meaning all was well, or answer the phone, giving me the opportunity to "respond to a crisis" on the other end of the line.

My phone rang.

I stared at it as it rang two times, trying to decide if I was going to be weak or strong.

It rang a third time.

I decided to be strong.

I answered the phone. I don't even remember what my friend said on the other end. This is what I said: "Oh, no, really? I'm sorry. I'll be right there." I hung up and told #11 the person on the phone was my son, who called to tell me he had a flat tire and I had to leave to rescue him. Which, if you knew me, you would know that, A) My son was still in school when he supposedly called, and B) he doesn't have a car.

Once safely out of the parking lot, I headed home and fell apart, and I remained there—apart—for a good few hours. I must have landed on my living room couch, playing the song "Keep Breathing" by Ingrid Michaelson about fifteen times in a row as I laid there, intermittently sobbing and pissed and exhausted, and pissed and sobbing. Oy. See, I'm not *that* strong!! I had not had a moment like that in months—*months,* I tell you! I have been so surrounded by positive attitudes and visualizations of nerve health and good outcomes and have been so grounded and calm that this really knocked me for a loop. I should have trusted my gut. I knew better. I knew this was going to happen and yet, I felt like I sort of let it happen. Maybe for a reason?

What came of this was yet another lesson for me. Right now, I need to take better care of myself. As if the last year wasn't enough! Right now, I need to protect myself better from well-meaning strangers and friends whose intentions may not be to scare me or challenge my process, but whose actions can and do. Right now, I need to surround myself with friends who will unconditionally support and love and nurture me. I feel so self-centered, it's a little nauseating. I urge you to do the same. Whether pre-surgery or not.

Why do we choose to have people in our lives who offer us anything less? There are plenty of relationships we have little or no choice over, right? Our boss, our next door neighbor, our coworkers. My point is that we can take care of ourselves, and we can surround ourselves with friends and family who are unconditionally on our team. We should nurture the relationships with people who will be there when we need them the very most, as well as when it's just another lazy, boring, obligation-free Saturday on the calendar.

COMMENTS

Bonnie has survived cancer. Twice. But more than that, she is the first friend I made by stalking. I first heard of her when she was on a local radio station, then she got in trouble for making a joke on the air. It was a joke similar to the one that got me fired from my job here in Bellingham. I knew I had to meet her, and then, one day, our mutual friend introduced us. I was so in awe of her, I could barely speak. I got over it eventually, and am lucky enough to consider her a friend now.

BONNIE said: I call people like #11 the vampires, Marla. They thrive on darkness and drama, sucking the good out of anyone who will give them a chance. Time is precious. Get the garlic!

LaVera is an artist, a mom, a friend. We met ten years ago in a mom's and friends group. She understands loss, and is very wise.

LAVERA said: Try to stay in the moment. Don't think so much about the future. You can deal with anything that comes your way as it comes, but you cannot control what has not happened, so don't try to.

SHIRLEY said: You and I know how strong you are, and I know that whatever the outcome, you will deal with it. But in my heart I know that the results will be good, and don't let yourself think otherwise. Whoever that gal was, I don't like her. She had NO RIGHT TO MAKE YOU THINK OTHERWISE BECAUSE YOU HAVE THE BEST DOCTORS AND EVERYONE IS THINKING POSITIVE. I LOVE YOU. MOM

My response: I love you too mom…

I'm hoping my outcome is as good as Adrienne's. I hope I can be the beacon of hope for someone else that she has been for me.

ADRIENNE said: I soooo know what you mean about people "sharing" too much. And that's helping, how??? Can't wait until you're on the other side and can share your POSITIVE OUTCOME story with whomever might need it in the future. After all, you can never hear enough from those with great outcomes, right? I wanted to hear more, more, more!

Two friends started a support group here in town, in response to their family members' cancer diagnoses. The special thing about this group is their name,"Flamingos and Friends." To show support to a person (and that person's family, for that matter) who is either in the early stages, in treatment, in remission, or doing anything else related to his or her diagnosis, the group will "flock" their front yard with hundreds of, you guessed it, pink flamingos. They raise money by people donating to have someone they know flocked. The flockings are seen around town throughout the year. Here is their Facebook page, in case you are interested:

https://www.facebook.com/pages/Flamingos-and-Friends/286850403947

February 8, 2010: Two and a wake up

Sunday morning I receive a surprise I certainly never expected. I step out my front door shortly after 7:00 AM to go for one of my last morning walks before surgery. To my surprise and shock … I have been FLOCKED!!

It takes my breath away, and then I notice heart shapes tied around the neck of each and every flamingo. I bend down to look at one, and it is a note from my sister Tara that she had posted on my online journal. And another note from another friend. I quickly determine, Norman or not, that these ladies have painstakingly printed what looks like every single blog comment posted on my online journal and then painstakingly cut and pasted each one onto a heart tied around the necks of each and every flamingo. It was then that the tears started.

There are few reasons this strikes me in such a profound manner. First, I don't have cancer. Second, I do not have a reputation in town for being a big money donor when it comes to non-profits. And third, I have no idea how I ever became worthy of the capacity for love and support this community has given to me over the past few months. For this and more, I am eternally grateful and humbled.

This day is a big day. I have mentioned the spiritual conditioning I have been doing. Acupuncture is in that category, as is my work with Dudley. I continue to feel healthy and grounded and clear and ready since working with her Saturday, and I even slept well every night since that night! Today I have an opportunity to do more work on that front with an intimate "Healing Ceremony" at my house with a handful of friends and family. This ceremony is with a few Jewish friends, some Christian friends, a few Unitarians, some random spiritualists, and even an agnostic. They are being called to be my "first line" prayer-and-positive-thought group, because they believe in it. Some more than others, most more than I. I'm covering all my bases. Never underestimate the power of positive thinking, right?

Oh. My. God. What if, what if, what if …

That just has to be enough today.

COMMENTS

Buff is a friend who moved out of state early in this process and kept up with my status. Her comments of support, and the rest of these below, including the one from my mom validated all of my hard emotional work.

BUFF said: What if everything goes right for you … just like everything you have done for and with friends has obviously gone very, very right? What if the doctors are on top of their game, as usual, and look inside your very wonderful head and take out everything that doesn't belong there. What if you wake up, just a tad groggy from the anesthesia, and find that people who love you are all teary because it all went right???? What if … what if … what if all your worries are just worries, and the reality is that you've arranged for the best … and you're the best, and everything will be all right? What if it's Thursday and you're eating Jell-O and waiting for discharge … what if you now have more free time and more energy to do more for and with friends and family …

Sally, a friend from community theater, who makes me laugh so hard I can sometimes barely control myself, knows me better than I thought. Truly a milestone!

SALLY said: Milestones in knowing you can't control everything!!!

Marilyn is my neighbor.

MARILYN said: Feeding the flamingos positive energy every time I drive by. Great to see the love and support.

TARA said: Life is full of what ifs. We can't control everything, which is so frustrating. Take a deep breath and love each day and appreciate it for the fact that we have it. Love the flocking, thank you Bellingham.

SHIRLEY said: I love you. Mom

My response: I love you too.

Chapter 4. PRE-OP

February 8, 2010: Miles to go before I sleep
What a day! I didn't have enough time for a full-on walk or a walking buddy this morning, but I made sure I got in a half hour around Zuanich Point Park, a lovely 2.6 mile walk—it is and will always be a great way to start the day.

Then it is down to Virginia Mason Hospital ... Pre-op should really be called TMI Overload. Thank goodness my friend and former health care provider Nancy is there with me, translating, asking the deeper questions, checking my face to make sure I am still breathing, which I am, thank you very much! We walk in and are greeted by a lovely woman who says to me, "You can't be the patient, you look too good!" Every positive comment helps. We go up to Neurosurgery, where we meet Dr. Farrokhi, who I will from now on refer to as Dr. Wonderful. He is very kind and just asks me what I want to know. I ask him a few superficial questions, which he answers gently, and then, I take a deep breath and, not knowing where the voice comes from but realizing it is mine, I say, "Okay, walk me through the day of surgery." Yeah. That came out of my mouth. Me, the one who doesn't usually want all the gory details. He calmly and again gently explains the IVs, the Spinal, the hair shaving, the neck muscle moving, the skull carving, the cerebellum moving, the tumor reduction, the nerve monitoring, the skull plugging and patching, the muscle relayering, the stitching, the recovery room. Yes, still breathing ...

Nancy asks him about the anticipated stay in the hospital. Remember, almost all of the former patients I have spoken with spent about six or seven days in the hospital. He says he had one patient who went home the next day, and she was seventy-two years old. The longest stay? Ten days, and it was a young woman who was an aerobics instructor. See? Being healthy is bad for you! (wink) So I am figuring my stay will be somewhere in between there. An informal pool was started yesterday. Big money is on me being home after four days.

I feel pretty good, then just as I thought he was done talking and I was done listening, he says, oh, now I need you to know all the possible things that can go wrong with this kind of surgery. Part of me screams, *Please, stop! I am focusing on the positive. I do not want or need to hear this!* But apparently I only scream it in my head because he tells me anyway. I know he has to tell me because of all of the informed consent rules, but I am not going to share them here. You don't need to hear them from me. There are plenty of online forums where you can get these horror stories. Or, better yet, you should hear them from your own doctor. I don't need to repeat it, and to be quite honest, I am back in the state of calm.

I ask him what they do with the tumor matter. He tells me, as I thought, they send if off to pathology to make sure it's not cancer, and then dispose of the rest. I guess, being a neurosurgeon, he has a lot of experience with brains, but I have no idea he can read minds because the next thing he says is, "No, you can't have the tumor to take home."

Me: "Why not?"

He says, "Because it came out of your body, and it's considered biohazard."

"Well, my kids came out of my body, and they let me take them home!"

He does not think that is as funny as I do.

So for the next little while, I sign the sanctity and safety of my life into the hands of this trusted doctor, and then I go over to pre-op anesthesia to meet the anesthesiologist. They tell me my heart and lungs are strong, I appear to be in great health, and I should bounce back just fine.

When I had my one and only other major surgery almost ten years ago, I read a book called *Prepare Yourself for Surgery,* by Peggy Huddleston. It is a great book, a kind of woo-woo book, and it comes with a tape that I listened to a number of times. It is about relaxation, visualization, and healing. I talked to my OBGYN surgeon about it, but she had never heard of it. She agreed to participate in the verbal exercises in the book the morning of my surgery, and she told me later that she had never seen a person bounce back from surgery that quickly.

I have been thinking about that for the past few days, and I ask the anesthesiologist if he will agree to participate in the "pre-surgery suggestive statement," and he says yes. This is my note to the doctors and nurses and the healing statements I'm asking them to say:

Dear doctors and nurses,

In preparation for my retrosigmoid surgery, I have prepared the following Healing Statements. Please read them to me at the times indicated. Please read the statements more than once (up to five times), and repeat them if you are interrupted or if anything remarkable happens in the room while you are reading the statements. Thank you so much. I hope that these statements will provide me with relaxation and comfort during and after the procedure.

Prior to Surgery / As I am going "under" statement:
You will relax completely. You will feel comfortable before, during, and after surgery. Your surgery will go well, and you will heal quickly afterward. Your tumor will be removed successfully, and your facial nerve will remain intact.

After Surgery statement:
Your operation has gone well! Your facial nerve is intact! You will heal promptly and feel comfortable. You will rest and awaken when you are ready.

In ICU statement:
Your facial nerve is intact. You are comfortable now, and you will awaken as if you had been asleep overnight, feeling rested. You will feel well, and you will remain calm. You will heal promptly and well.

Thank you so much! Please feel free to say other positive, healing, and peaceful statements to me.
—*Marla Bronstein*

I think this is the last bit of control and planning and organizing I have done to prepare for surgery.

This has been my plan all along.

I'm home later, and I'm folding towels from the laundry and thinking, "Hmm, I really don't feel that different at all after the surgery." As if it's over already and I'm already recovered. All that happens unintentionally. But I like it. And I will keep that feeling of "It's already over, I feel pretty darn good!" So informed consent or not, I plan to get out of there in one piece, sans Norman.

February 9, 2010: Have faith. Don't buy the flight insurance

We are in Seattle. My sister Tara, my friend Nancy who came with me yesterday for my pre-op, and my friend Alyssa are all here tonight. Tomorrow, I check in at 5:30 AM, and my surgery starts at 7:30 AM. I decide they will be done in about four hours, and I will go home Saturday. Hearing and facial nerve intact. Just in case you were curious.

Have Faith. Don't buy the flight insurance. That's the whisper my friend Jana said to me. Have faith. Believe in the doctors, the hospital, the treatment, the planning and preparation, the care-givers, the supporters, the well wishers, and all of you reading this and holding me today and in the days past and in the days to come.

I walked the waterfront this morning ... it was blanketed in fog. I knew the water was there, I knew the islands, the barges, the boats that have been trolling for the past few weeks were all there, but I couldn't see them. I just knew they were there. Like I can't "see" Thursday, but I know it will be there. And it will be just as I know it to be now ... a new Norman-less Normal.

Before I go in for surgery, I do not say goodbye. Before I go in for surgery, I do not write any of those letters you want to write or are supposed to write when you think your life might be over soon and you have things to say you don't want to be left unsaid. Before I go in for surgery, I do not finish my sewing projects. I do not make Caleb's high school graduation book. I do not finish the laundry, make a ton of food for the freezer, plant flowers for spring, or arrange for the furnace to be serviced. I have faith.

I have chosen the best doctors, the best facility, the best procedure for me. I have prepared myself physically and mentally for a successful surgery. I have controlled everything I have had any possible amount of control over, and tomorrow morning at seven-thirty, I will let all that go and give it up to the team. Now if they all just do their job ... it will all be fine, right? Right!

And I did not buy the flight insurance.

Chapter 5. WAITING, WAITING, WAITING

The next few days of entries were written by Ken, Tara, and Alyssa. I had to give up all control and had to not worry or think or consider anyone else for the almost ten hours the doctors had my life in their hands. There were hundreds of comments and words of support, encouragement, and love left in this short span of days. I'm sure that's the main reason I am here to share this story with you. I have only included two poems for your enjoyment.

February 10, 2010 7:24 AM: And it begins

This is Ken writing from the waiting room at Virginia Mason Hospital. Marla spent the night at a hotel in Seattle near the hospital, with her sister Tara and good friend Nancy. Alyssa stayed with a friend in town. She arrived with her entourage at VM for her 5:30 AM check-in, and I arrived shortly thereafter, having driven down from Bellingham early in the morning.

Marla was in good spirits as we waited for her to start the check-in process. They finally called her to get her lovely ID bracelets and to take more information, in preparation to lead her upstairs to surgery prep. At about six-fifteen, a very nice orderly dressed in scrubs called Marla's name. He led her to the elevator and was very patient as we said our goodbyes. We were all quite teary-eyed as we hugged and said words of love and support. Then she entered the elevator to begin the solo journey.

We were given a beeper, just like the ones you get when waiting for a table at a restaurant. This will be used to inform us as she reaches certain milestones, like surgery start, surgery end, headed for recovery, etc. There is also an electronic reader board, which lists these milestones for all patients. Everyone is assigned a number upon check-in. Marla is 21080. So we can follow the scrolling messages and watch for updates.

Currently, Marla's status is "in surgery prep." We expect that the surgery will start about seven thirty. We are expecting that the surgery will take six to eight hours, not including about a one-hour prep.

That's all for now.

9:02 AM: In the doctor's hands

Marla's surgery has started. Tara, Nancy and I are taking a ten-minute break to send love and positive thoughts into the operating room about the surgery and recovery. The positive energy and love sent by all of you is greatly appreciated. Many are even lighting candles. Marla will really appreciate that as well, as she is a believer in lighting candles for any occasion (especially Chanukah, as you may have figured out!).

11:28 AM: Waiting

So it turns out that when they told me Marla was "in surgery," she was just moved into the OR. The first incision took place at nine fifteen. That's over two hours of prep!

This place has twenty-four operating rooms (I forget the actual term they use ... studios?). There are a lot of people here in the waiting area, and occasionally a doctor comes out after a patient is done and speaks with the family/friends. Nice to see that happening, and I think I speak for my whole "team" here when I say we look forward to the time the doc comes out to do the same with us.

So much great energy coming this way! Thank you! I'm wiping away a little tear (or two or three) every time I read a comment or get a text that someone has lit a candle, or is sending energy, or praying for Marla. Both kids told me that they have permission to take calls, even at school or work, reminding me that there are many people who I may not even know of who are keeping Marla in their thoughts.

I envision that, about now, Norman is being dislodged from the site where he has been trespassing for so long. About time!

1:39 PM: No news is good news

Marla has been in surgery (in the surgical suite, as Tara corrects me) for over four hours now. That is the amount of time that the doctors said was the minimum her surgery would take. At this point we are fairly certain that Norman has been evicted, leaving more room in Marla's head for even more great comebacks, inspired ideas, and whatever else strikes her fancy. Nancy is betting on six hours. Maybe we should have a pool going.

While the waiting room is still pretty busy, recently a bunch of surgeries have finished, and the doctors have come to meet with families. We were about the first here, and we will be here probably quite a bit longer. But the time is going quickly. We're reading, working (that's me!), eating lunch, listening to music (me again), and chatting. Tara got a journal, and we've all contributed our thoughts, so Marla can read it later on and experience her surgery from another angle.

Thanks for all of the posts, Facebook comments, and texts. I even got a call from someone who isn't on the blog or Facebook to express his support. I told Marla (in the journal) that I get to bask in the love and good energy coming her way. It is wonderful. Thank you all.

2:54 PM: New sheriff in town

We know now that the big guns are working together to make sure Norman gets out and stays out. We just heard a page in the waiting room for "family of John Wayne." We all, very inappropriately, broke out laughing. But if that's the kind of backup the wonderful doctors have called in, more power to them!

Okay, we're getting a little punchy. We sent Nancy out for a game ... cards, Scrabble, something to keep us from acting up in this very public setting. I'm sure Marla would be plotting something even more entertaining. She'll be with us soon, I know. It is nearly six hours since surgery started. About an hour or so ago, Tara asked at the desk how it was going, and they called upstairs to the surgery receptionist. We were assured that everything was going very well, Marla was doing fine, but they still had a couple of hours to go. Hopefully she'll be done before the four of us cause any serious trouble!

This was from my friend Barbara, to my faithful posse:

In the spirit of preserving your sanity, and supporting your endurance:

The Clown Chakra

The Clown Scientists have found that all our problems can be placed under one heading: Seriousness. Seriousness is the leading cause of everything from Cancer to Reincarnation. Scientists from the Clown Academy have already discovered a new source of healing.
It is a psychic energy point located between the heart chakra and the throat chakra.
It is called the Clown Chakra.
If people are feeling miserable,
if they have financial problems,
if their relationship situation is the pits,
if they are in ill health,
if they have a need to sue people,
if they find fault with their brother,
then obviously,

their Clown Chakra is closed.

When this happens,

the scientists have observed under a high-powered microscope that the cells of every organ display a sad face, and when the Clown Chakra is open and functioning normally, the cells display a happy face. The scientists realized that if a person is ill, it is because his mind has projected guilt onto the cells of his body and has forced out the love that is normally found within each cell of the body.

The cells are therefore saying,

"I Lack Love," or "ILL" for short.

The scientists also discovered that all disease is due to the fact that the cells are out of ease or dis-eased.

When the Clown Chakra is opened and working (or rather, playing) properly,

the psychic mechanism sucks up misery, pain, anger, resentment, grievances, unhappiness, etc., and converts the energy into tiny red heart-shaped balloons.

The red heart-shaped balloons contain Love and Joy.

These balloons are directed to the dis-eased cell or situation, and a happy face appears instantly.

When the light enters the darkness, the darkness is gone.

Sometimes these red heart-shaped balloons are called endorphins,

due to the fact that when anyone experiences them, the feeling of separation ends.

They experience being back home with All That Is and hence are no longer an orphan.

This is the well-known end-orphan (endorphin) effect.

So, if you think someone is attacking you,

Clown Scientists recommend that you visualize sending that person red heart-shaped balloons filled with Love and Joy.

Remember to keep your Clown Chakra open and remember to laugh.

Seriousness causes reincarnation.

3:31 PM: Closing time

We were just visited by Marla's ENT, Dr. Backous. The surgery is done, and Dr. Farrokhi is now closing. About an hour and she's out.

The news Dr. Backous had wasn't as good as we had hoped. Marla came out of it just fine, and she is in no danger. But Norman was very, very tenacious. In fact, they left a small amount of tumor, for fear of damaging Marla's facial nerve. He said the tumor had stretched the nerve about two centimeters, which is miles for a nerve. The readings for nerve response were good, but due to the stretching and the manipulation from the surgery, he wasn't sure what the end result of her facial nerve function would be. He said it could take up to nine months for the nerve to recover.

They will monitor the tumor remains and see what happens. There's no threat that they'll have to go back in. If there's growth, they can radiate effectively. He said out of ten times they've had to leave some of the tumor behind, only in two cases has there been growth. Sometimes it actually shrinks.

So we're not out of the woods yet. Your positive thoughts, good energy, prayers, are still needed. We'll be speaking with Dr. Farrokhi in a few minutes and see if he has any new information. And then we'll get to see Marla, once she wakes up. There's still lots to do, but I am confident Marla has the team behind her to support her through whatever her recovery will look like.

I can't wait for her to see the wonderful, supportive comments you have all made on this blog.

5:24 PM: Good riddance, Norman!

We had a wonderful, informative meeting with the neurosurgeon, Dr. Farrokhi. We learned a lot about our old nemesis. Norman had grown aggressively in the two months since the last MRI. Plus, he was the consistency of a sticky marshmallow. The tumor peeled off of the brain stem easily (that's hugely important). But it was very, very involved with the facial nerve.

So a tiny amount was left behind, rather than risk more damage to the facial nerve.

All of the major issues surrounding this surgery went very well. Marla tolerated the anesthesia very well, and she was very stable throughout this very long, invasive procedure. The questions remaining have to do with the possibility of lasting damage to the facial nerve, and whether Marla will have any residual hearing. As far as the hearing, Dr. Farrokhi gave it a 50/50 chance (which is much better than we had originally expected). The facial nerve is harder to tell. A lot of that has to do with the next twenty-four hours and how well the swelling is controlled. The readings of the nerve were the same before and after the surgery. So we are very, very hopeful.

Norman was sent to pathology, and we won't know the results for five to seven days. The chances of malignancy are very small, but always present.

Both doctors had wonderful bedside manners. Dr. Farrokhi talked about the affirmations that Marla had given him and his crew to read throughout the surgery. He normally does that during surgery, and he was more than happy to say very positive, affirmative things while Marla was unconscious. The doctor spent a good amount of time with the now five of us (Marla's friend Kathy showed up too) and answered in lots of detail the lay person's questions (mine), and well as the professional medical providers' questions. We all feel very optimistic that, despite the tenacity and aggressiveness of Norman, the absolute best team was in place, and Marla can expect the absolute best outcome under the circumstances.

We'll get to see her in about an hour. Tomorrow we'll know much more about how well she is and how well she will recover from this. Hopefully tomorrow will be my last day as the scribe for this blog, and the originator herself will re-take her rightful position as the blog poster. Thanks for all of your wonderful comments. It is an honor to have you all in our circle of friends and supporters.

9:50 PM: Start to heal

After our meeting with Farrokh (his first name, by which he always introduces himself), we had to wait for Marla to get released from recovery, have a CAT scan, and then get settled into her room in the ICU (it is actually the ICU overflow, as the regular ICU is full!). We went up to see her and were first told she needed more time to settle in. After about fifteen or twenty minutes, we were told that she didn't want to see anyone and that she said she needed at least another twenty minutes. This was hard to take, especially for Tara, who came to Seattle specifically to be with Marla when she was at her most vulnerable. Well, it turns out that Marla was feeling extremely nauseous (not a surprise, under the circumstances). If you know Marla, you know that nausea is her least favorite feeling in the world! And she didn't want anyone to see her in that condition. So after about a total of thirty minutes, she was feeling better, and Tara and I went in to see her.

She looked exhausted, but beautiful. And Tara even got her to smile (yes, both sides of the mouth did respond!) Then Nancy, Alyssa, and Kathy came in for very short visits. Tara is going to stay overnight with her in the ICU. Hopefully there will be a whole lot of sleeping going on tonight, especially in that ICU room.

I am staying at my dear friend Rennie's house in Wallingford, Nancy had to head back to Bellingham, and Alyssa is staying with a friend in Seattle. Alyssa and I will re-convene at Virginia Mason in the morning, and hopefully Marla will be less nauseous, less tired, and ready to start the hard work of recovery. She will be visited by both doctors and will get up and take a little walk. She is also scheduled for a Norman postmortem MRI.

We'll probably start to get a feel for how long she might need to recover at that point. Nausea and dizziness are the prime indications that she is not ready to go home. If, as we hopefully expect, she is well along the road to adjusting to living without the left vestibular nerve, she could be on the way home sooner rather than later. It just remains to be seen.

It has been a treat and privilege to be the official Marla blogger today. As much as I have enjoyed it, I hope to be relieved of this duty sooner rather than later. Whatever happens, I'm sure we will keep you informed.

February 11, 2010, 9:30 AM: The day after (by Ken)

I spent the night at my friend's house in Seattle and stayed in touch with the events at the hospital by texting Tara. Marla got some sleep, even though she was woken up often for neurological tests. Tara got a few hours of sleep as well! Marla is still feeling a bit nauseous, for which she is receiving medication, but she has had no headaches.

She was visited by Farrokh early this morning, who said she looks better than most of his patients at this stage. She has good facial response and eye squint. She is going in for the MRI this morning, which should shed more light on where she is following the surgery. She'll also be visited by Dr. Backous.

Marla commented to Farrokh that she thought she could hear a bit out of her left ear. The doctor said it could take up to three months to know whether that hearing will be preserved or not.

I'm about to head over to the hospital now and will report any new information when I get it.

1:17 PM: Moving day

Hi, this is Tara, Marla's sister. I am excited to tell you that Marla is moving out of the ICU up to the neurosurgical floor. She is off her blood pressure meds and will try eating some clear liquids shortly. Her MRI looked good—no bleeding or swelling! This was the "Get out of Jail Free" card! Physical Therapy was here, and she was able to stand and side step with very minimal nausea. She did these funky eye exercises where she had to follow a pen with her eyes up and down and at a diagonal for a minute each in four different directions. It made me nauseated! The physician assistants for Dr. Farrokhi stopped by to meet with us, and they were very impressed with Marla and the way she is

81

improving—they loved the way the anesthesiologist spoke her positive affirmations. They said he really said it from the heart. They also said they would like to see that more in the OR.

I have always known that my sister is a very special person—kind, caring, and giving—but the way her friends and family have supported her have confirmed it even more. I would like to thank you all for everything you have done so far, and for what I know you all plan on doing in the future. I know you all are worried about her facial nerve, but when I saw her smile after surgery, I had to hold back my tears, knowing that her facial nerve is safe and that she will smile, walk, and be the same quick-witted person she always has been.

Ken went back home to bring Caleb back to see his mom and visit with his best friend. Marla has kept her sense of humor and is taking a lot of naps. We are all looking forward to a peaceful evening with another visit from physical therapy (PT) and occupational therapy (OT), and hopefully in the next day or so, we will have a clearer idea of when we get to bring her home and how the rest of her recuperation will go. Inch by inch, then mile by mile!

5:42 PM: View from the seventeenth floor

Alyssa ("Moodypants"!) here to update you, live from Marla's new room!

After a brief lunch break off campus, Tara and I returned to find both PT and OT were ready for round two with our sweet Marla. In spite of the fact that she is still a bit groggy from all the activity and medications, with a bit of assistance and guidance, she was able to walk an entire loop around the unit and transfer into her new bed before we moved her upstairs. Now she is settled, and once again resting comfortably. We are still hearing from her hospital caregivers that her recuperation is going very, very well. She's moving herself around in bed and chatting with us when awake. She is still on a clear liquid diet, but we are hoping for an upgrade soon! We are steadily getting her back to the Marla we all know and love.

Thank you all SO MUCH for the constant stream of wonderful messages you continue to post. Know that we are always checking for new ones and reading them to Marla, so she isn't missing a single, wonderful word everyone is sharing.

Tara and I are holding down the fort while we wait for Ken to return with Caleb for the evening. Tonight we rest in preparation for more PT and OT and plotting and scheming our return trip home with Marla, sans Norman.

This in response from my friend Gwen:

GWEN said:

"Ode to Norman"
Bye bye, Norman, you ugly creep who had a wretched grip on our Marla
You've released your hold, HA—you were not so bold—She's proven to be much stronga
Your arrogant grip led us all on a trip,
We thought you a powerful fellow
Only to find out that for all your clout you were weak as a spongy marshmallow
You'll not be missed, and although we're pissed
That you put Marla and us through your hell.
You've been evicted (as love, courage, and skill predicted)
AND OUR MARLA WILL SOON BE WELL!

February 12, 2010, noon: Heading into new normal
We don't know where to begin ... (co-written by Tara, Alyssa, and Ken):

Dr. Wonderful (Farrokh) came by at seven thirty this morning to say Marla should be ready to go home by tonight or tomorrow! Needless to say, we were shocked! We literally wanted to jump out of our seats. He was full of information: Only a few of Norman's remains were still on the facial nerve, and they were much smaller than they had originally thought. A "hot spot" on the MRI, which can indicate that there had been a stroke, turns out to be the result of where the retractor was during surgery. Marla also passed other tests, like following the doctor's finger, reaching to touch his finger, and then touching her nose (interesting test!); all those tests showed that there was no danger she had suffered a stroke!

He gave her many positive comments; all were great to hear. He also said that when the steroids that she is taking to reduce brain swelling are stopped, the facial swelling may reappear, but it will most likely gradually decrease on its own—hopefully any deficit we would see is temporary.

Later, Dr. Superman (Backous) stopped by with more positive things to say! The preliminary biopsy of Norman was benign, which we expected. He also said there seems to be no more swelling, and he thinks that she is safe to discharge to go home tomorrow morning, erring on the side of caution by keeping her an extra night. That will provide her a bit more rest and PT and OT so that Marla feels stronger when she gets back to Bellingham. She will, of course, still be quite tired when she does get back and will absolutely need all the rest she can get … but we all know her recuperation will increase exponentially when she is back in her own bed surrounded by even more people that adore her.

This is from Tara (Nurse Ratched):
Today we have a list of goals for what is going to be a very busy day: She will take a shower, go for another walk, do more PT and OT, try out the stairs (we're on the seventeenth floor, but we doubt she'll go too far!), and get more sleep. Things we now try to avoid include constipation, blood clots, and pneumonia. We know that none of these things are going to happen. She is up moving, taking deep breaths, and drinking prune juice. Physical therapy is here now doing her vestibular nerve tracking exercises. Marla is making jokes, and instead of laughing I get choked up. She will be up and about before we know it. I can

imagine her feeling better and wanting to do more once she has been home, the overachiever she is.

She had a good night's sleep, and she got up to go to the bathroom a few times. Shared room issues did present themselves. The woman in then next bed had some kidney problems, so I called her "Mrs. Nephrectomy." She was upset when we got up at 2:00 AM because we had to turn on the lights to get to the bathroom safely. I left Marla in the bathroom and went down the hall so we could both have empty bladders, and when I got back, Marla was getting yelled at by Mrs. Nephrectomy! "I know you are sick, but I am too, and I need rest." Of course, I felt absolutely horrible that we had bothered her; it's the last thing I wanted to do. Marla said nothing. The nurse came in and did vital signs and her hourly neurological check, which consisted of smiling, puffing up her cheeks, squeezing her fingers, and asking her name and date of birth. Then it was lights off so we could all go back to sleep.

Around six-fifteen this morning, Mrs. Nephrectomy's doctor came in and asked how she was feeling. She complained about us talking and kids screaming in the hallway, and how we were up in middle of night, and we had visitors late she went to sleep at seven-thirty (and we didn't). Then her doctor said her kidney cancer was all removed and she would rest better at home. We are happy for her, and especially that she will be discharged today. Proximity always adds to the excitement. Also, how do non-private rooms fit in the line of HIPPA protocol? Even though I loved The Bucket List, I have yet to see a good roommate situation.

Marla has now finished her walk, is still having dizziness and some pain, but is back in bed sleeping soundly. We are doing stairs this afternoon.

When Marla was up in the chair, we put her laptop in front of her, but then breakfast showed up (solid food!). She is not ready yet, but soon will take over this blog.

I have loved your comments. I read them to Marla while she is lying in bed. We all love it.

Chapter 6. NORMAN DOESN'T LIVE HERE ANYMORE

Three days after my surgery, I was "forced" to write in my journal. It was slow going, but I had missed it, so it felt good. I tried to remember everything, I'm sure I didn't. For the purposes of clarification, the pen the doctors used for the funky eye test was dubbed "Tiki Man" because it had a Tiki Torch carved face where the eraser part should have been. I was supposed to track his head with my eyes and not move my head. This was part of the vestibular exercise I did three or four times each day, to help me regain my balance.

Here's what I was able to piece together from the time they carted me in to the surgery prep area.

February 13, 2010: Taking back control ... sort of
The moment I get called to go in for my surgery prep, it feels a little like Dead Man Walking, and saying goodbye to my family and friends scares the crap out of me. Having Ken, Tara, Alyssa, and Nancy holding and hugging me for luck and support is so amazing. The nurse, David, is very reassuring and brings me back to the area to change into my surgery garb. A very nice nurse helps me attach a power stone from my friend Julie to one of my wristbands. Then Rusty, one of the anesthesia team, comes in to put in my first of many IVs. I show him my positive

affirmation letter, and he not only agrees to it, he also promises he will get everyone else in the operating room to do it too. Then Dr. Wonderful comes in looking as yuppie as possible and sharp, as if he is headed to a frat party. He also promises he will remain positive, and finally, Dr. Superman shows up in sweats. I ask him if he is working today, and he assures me he is and says he is on his way to meet my family. At this point I am sure they think I am some kind of woo-woo freak, but it all gives me comfort, and I know it was part of my surgery plan.

So there I sit for another half hour or so, waiting for someone to come take me back to where I need to be. I guess I am a little discombobulated because I remember Rusty coming back into the room but not much else. He warns me about going into the surgery room with the noises and the people and the lights, but honestly I don't remember any of that. I do have a very clear memory of him speaking the words of affirmation to me as I go under, and the next thing I remember is hearing him say the words of post surgery as I am I coming out of anesthesia and am being transported to recovery.

I have no idea how long it's been.

The first thing I do when I realize where I am is freeze.

I want to touch my face.

My hand feels like it weighs one hundred pounds.

I want to touch my face. My curiosity overtakes my greatest fear that I won't feel anything. That I'll have facial paralysis. That all the "right" things I did will be "wrong."

I want to touch my face. Slowly, with great effort, my left hand moves.

I just know if I can feel my face, I can move it.

Well, yes I do, and yes I can.

My left cheek, my lips, my left eye.

And I start to cry.

Well, sob really.

All of the work I had done, all of the research. Choosing the right doctors for me, the right facility. All of that brings me to where I am at this moment.

I lose all track of time. I know it was about five-ish when I got out of surgery only because I am so acclimated to finding clocks when I wake up. I know Tara wanted to sneak into recovery, she's done it before with my mom, but they are too good in this hospital, and they do not let anyone back to see me right away. Not until they are ready, and then not until I am ready. I am shaking badly as the anesthesia works its way out of my system. I calm myself using my meditation breathing I learned from Dudley. It clears out my lungs really well, and my lung function is excellent today.

Then the neuro checks start. Everyone asking me my name, the date, my date of birth, and the president. Smile. Puff my cheeks. Squint. Squeeze hands. Every hour. Every doctor, physical therapist, every nurse.

My night in ICU is not a fun night for anyone. As much as they warned me about the nausea, I think I am strong enough to control it. Which I do. With drug help after three in the morning. Until then I eat and drink nothing.

I am moved to another room the next day, where I actually stand up, walk around, eat food—well, clear liquids—and do my Tiki Man exercises thanks to Nurse Ratched.

I am going home tomorrow. Day four. I have yet to read all the comments that have come in, although some have been read to me. I am so grateful to all of you. Your comments, good wishes, and loving thoughts carried me to this place, and I will never forget the support and love you have given me. I have a long road ahead, and it has already started.

I had decided to make myself a poster of sorts to bring with me to the hospital and to have in my room there and for when I returned home. I have so many photos of myself with my friends who travelled with me on this journey of the past six months that mean so much to me. I get so much strength from my friends. One photo I took when I was in New York last fall, when I actually met Rosie

O'Donnell. I love that woman! I don't know why ... maybe it's because we are both big girls from Long Island.

Every day, then and now, I was and am, acutely aware of other people's struggles, and how mine were and are infinitesimal in comparison. The hospital staff loved my poster. They loved everything I brought with me—the heart notes that were wrapped around the pink flamingos, the photos ... they all ask me, "How do you know Rosie?" It's amazing this power of celebrity. (smile!)

February 14, 2010: And so the time of lessons to be learned begins

Tara ("Nurse Ratched") told me I have to write something today since you have all been so great standing by my side online, cheering me on, but to be quite honest, this is the hardest part of the journey for me. Not having my full abilities to do just about anything is frustrating, humbling, and annoying, and not necessarily in that order. Nurse Ratched gets mad when I don't let her know I am going to the bathroom.

Or getting dressed.

Or answering the phone.

In case I fall.

Whatever!

I am not supposed to lift anything heavier than a half gallon of milk. I wonder if I can get away with not doing laundry or going to the grocery store for a year? What a bonus that would be!

Tara is taking amazing care of us. She has organized the fridge, my room, and the shower, just so that I won't hurt myself. Things are moved so I don't have to bend over. Handles are placed in case I start to lose my balance. Furniture is moved so I don't have to walk around it. A shower chair is purchased so I don't fall down. Tomorrow she is "training" the women who have volunteered to take care of me when Ken and Caleb are at work and school. Again, it's a very hard place for me to find myself, but I am doing my best to recover from surgery. You only get one chance, you know? After that, you are recovering from all the stupid things you did when you thought you were all better and you weren't.

If you ever have to have surgery, major or minor, I hope you have someone like Tara in your corner. She has been here every step of the way (literally), and I could not/would not feel this confident and calm without her. I know she is leaving Tuesday (sigh), but her organization of my home and her attention to detail of every little thing I need to do, and that Ken and Caleb and the caregivers will need to do, has made all the difference in the world. Tara is my hero.

My friend Iris came over and fixed my hair today. Dr. Wonderful has great neurosurgical skills, but he apparently skipped the Vidal Sassoon lesson day of surgery school. Now it looks totally cute, a little bobbed and even on both sides. I get the surgical staples out Friday—there are nineteen. After that, I won't worry about burning my head with the blow dryer.

My list of what I need help doing is so long and ridiculous (getting my clothes ready for the day, getting a glass of water, picking something up from the floor, getting in and out of the shower), and I feel like a total invalid. I hate it. But I sort of know it's temporary and I will grow from this experience. I hate being so needy and helpless. Did I say hate? Maybe that's not a strong enough word. I mean I HATE it! This is not how I get along in life. But I am learning to ask for and accept help. And that is my lesson of the day.

February 15, 2010: Noon (minor) setback

This is Ken writing again, this time from St. Joe's Hospital in Bellingham. Marla gave us a good scare this morning at about 8:00 AM. She fainted in the bathroom, and we heard a thump as she hit the floor, and possibly the side of the bathtub. Tara was there immediately, and Marla came-to in a matter of seconds. I called 911, and in moments we were overrun with EMTs and paramedics.

Even though she seemed fine, they found her blood pressure very low, and they decided to send her to the ER at St. Joe's. She's been on an IV since she arrived, plus they gave her some pain meds. She had a CT scan, which showed no sign of bleeding, so they're releasing her very shortly.

The plan for the rest of the day is rest and sleep, followed by some more rest and sleep. This episode makes it very clear to us, and also to Marla, how careful we need to be in these early stages of her recovery. We've learned that we need to keep an even closer eye on her, and perhaps put in one or two more safety bars in the bathroom. And I think Marla learned to be more aware of her dizziness, and to not try to get up if she is particularly weak or dizzy. We will try to have a blood pressure cuff with her at all times and to monitor her blood pressure before she tries to mobilize.

So, short story is, Marla is still doing well. But we did get a rude wakeup call. Many of you who've been through a rehabilitation period have cautioned her about not overdoing it. Well, now I hope we know better what that looks like, and we'll all be more cautious.

———

I guess I spoke too soon about falling, huh? I was VERY careful again after my fall. I scared everyone pretty well, myself included. I don't think I ever fainted before this. I do remember standing up, feeling spinny, and I even remember starting to fall, but the actual fall felt like a dream. I probably shouldn't say this, but being aware of losing consciousness was really interesting in an I-wouldn't-totally-mind-doing-that-again-but-in-a-softer-landing-place way. Then I remember Tara standing over me, calling my name, and sadly, seeing Caleb behind her completely freaked out. She sat me up but would not let me stand up. Ken called 911 (seriously?), and the paramedics got to the house in seconds! By the way, I am kitty-corner from the fire station! I don't know why they needed sirens blaring, but, sigh, they did. Just wondering, to qualify to be a paramedic, do you have to look like a soap opera actor?

I was embarrassed, but they INSISTED on carrying me down the stairs. Oy again. And then they carried me into the ambulance and drove me ten blocks to the hospital. I'll fast-forward through the new MRI and all that other testing (which came out fine), but I do want to point out that it took Tara a LONG time to arrive to the hospital after we did. When I asked her what took her so long, I realized she had fixed her hair and put on make up. Did I mention the cute paramedics?

February 18, 2010: A week and a day
Wow.

That's all I can say about this journey this past week. And I can't say enough about my family and my friends. My mother wants you to know that she loves all of you. I bet you could get a meal and an overnight at her house if you play your cards right. Yeah, that's where I get it from.

My left hand is still slower than my right, the left side of my face still tingles, and the left side of my tongue is still numb, but I am so much happier than I thought I would be by today. You know how I need to be right, right? I was home Saturday—my vestibular nerve on the right had done a lot of compensating pre-surgery, enabling me to come home as early as I did; walking all those mornings gave me strength and endurance to get out of the hospital; and all the woo-woo positive thinking, affirmations, and visualization meditation calmed me from panic. And here I am.

Bored. Bored. Bored.

I know, right?

I am NOT complaining, believe me—I just forgot how to be bored.

I was not prepared to be bored. I don't know what I thought I would be. Tired? Dizzy? Comatose? Unconscious? After filling up the past six months with day and night activities to keep me distracted from freaking out, I feel like the escalator just ended and

I am still in a perpetual state of moving forward, with nowhere to go and the inability (for now) to go there. I had forsaken TV and trashy reading for months, thinking now would be the time I would have to do that, but it just makes me dizzy. And sleepy. I know I'm supposed to sleep, but even that is not a restful sleep.

There were a few other things I could have been more prepared for. I could have met with all the lovely women who are my caregivers before the surgery to show them around my house. I could have gotten the safety bars and chairs ready for the bathrooms. And I could have arranged for an upstairs and downstairs walker before. But I guess I didn't know I'd need them. I still don't know if everyone who has this surgery does. Well, you do now, right?

I remember when my mom was so sick a few years ago and we had to force feed her protein. I don't remember why she didn't eat. Was it her taste buds? Her appetite? She wasn't sick to her stomach; she just didn't like the hospital food. Come to think of it, if she did, we probably would have had to call for a psych check. Well, I have no appetite, and everything I have "taste memories" of does not taste like I remembered it. Strange. As my friend Ro says, this is not the time to diet. Trust me, dieting is not my plan, but I certainly do not want to come out of this needing a guest spot on a daytime talk show as the woman who could not get out the door without a crowbar. A happy medium would be fine.

Speaking of memories, the other day I woke up to whispers in my ear. They are there forever, and hopefully there will be more to be heard after the swelling goes down. If you didn't get to whisper in person but left me a message on my cell phone, know that I used that to put your voice in my head. Yes, even you mom. I love you too.

Feeling a bit grateful and overwhelmed at the support of the past six months ...

February 23, 2010: A personal love letter to you

Dear (fill in your name here),

I am writing this long overdue letter to you today. It's sort of an update, but mostly a thank you. For everything. For your kind words spoken and unspoken before my surgery, for your comments on this blog, written and unwritten, for you cards purchased and not purchased, sent and unsent, and for your continued concern. I know you followed me through surgery. I felt you there with me the night before and the morning of, and as I waited in pre-op, I felt you with me, wishing me well, hanging on to faith that it was the right thing at the right time.

When I woke up after surgery, you were the first person I wanted to call, but I couldn't—obviously, I was in no shape to make phone calls. When I finally wrestled this journal back to post my own comments, I wanted to tell you how much I appreciated everything you wrote, I have read every word, but admit for some of it I was still under medication. I will take the opportunity in the next few days to really relish the time you took to reach out to me. And know that just because you may not have written as much as someone else, I can tell when you logged on, so I know you were there. (Tell me you are surprised I am part stalker. I have made some of my dearest friends by stalking them.)

I have had a couple of outings. I am going to try to go for a real walk outside on Friday and maybe even go to a play or two and a birthday party this weekend. No promises. Taking things day by day, not pushing myself too much, but I miss the world and you, my friend, so much. I can never repay you for the gift you have been to me for the past months. Know how much I love you, and if you ever need me, I will be there for you in whatever way I can be.

Love, Marla

I am just finishing my second week post-surgery. The majority of the light-headedness is gone. I am not half as dizzy as I was, although I still walk a little like a sailor at port after a few too many cocktails. When I walk, I am more stable with walls around or a shoulder or arm to hang on to. I graduated myself from needing-a-walker status after watching an old man cross the street slowly with his. Still don't have a great appetite for much healthy food. I have been happily "choking" down homemade chocolate chip cookies and the best noodle kugel ever. I guess my sweet taste buds are working the best. I have a funny taste in my mouth all the time, like I have been sucking on an old sweater. Yum. But do not hear me complaining at all.

Last Friday was the day I was scheduled to go to Seattle to have the nineteen staples removed, which the nurse did without incident. Nothing leaked out, like spinal fluid or any other fluid that wasn't supposed to that day or since. The incision site has nicely scabbed over and occasionally itches, which is a good healing sign, right? Dr. Wonderful came in and looked at the wound and was really pleased and asked me if I was happy for the outcome. HAPPY? I am the poster child for happy. I am doing what the doctor says and washing it every day, with no (or very minimal) hair product. Since I can't dye my hair for a while, as the gray grows in, I should look like Witchy Witch by March 11, when I am scheduled for my one-month follow-up.

The swelling is going down on the surgical site as well, and I can sort of feel where they drilled the hole. It's kind of strange, and magical also, to feel my skull healing. The body is an amazing thing. I will never take my health for granted again. I don't take much of the pain meds, only as needed about every other day or so. I wait until I think it will keep me from sleeping or eating or whatever I have to do. And I have been told I only have to rest right now. How odd is that for me? I have no resting skills.

March 2, 2010: Cold turkey

After getting more than ten updates the day of my surgery, and then hearing about me almost daily after that, I thought you would want a break from the day-by-day. Today we heard from a relative who was annoyed that she had no idea what was

95

going on anymore. Pardon me from trying to spare you from the mundane that is my life these days. Here you go:

Wake up. Take Tylenol. Check Facebook. Shower. Fix my hair. Eat breakfast. Check Facebook. Do Tiki-Man exercises. Check Facebook. Go for walk and/or lunch and/or tea. Come home. Check Facebook. Nap. Wake up. Check Facebook. (Yeah, I know I have a problem.) Watch TV or movie online. Check Facebook. Take Tylenol. Go to sleep. Wake up. Repeat.

See? It's boring. I don't have the patience to read anything like a book or even a magazine article right now. I'm so out of the habit of reading anything longer than a social media status or comment. Sad, pathetic me. I have quite a life these days.

But truly, I am not at all miserable, other than feeling like I am in jail in my own home. Jail with better clothes. My jailers are my friends—they do encourage me to get out of the house, but I am never allowed to be alone. I am looking forward to seeing my doctors for my one-month follow-up next week. I want them to give me permission to live independently again, without 24/7 care. I still don't have any hearing in my left ear, but the swelling seems to have subsided substantially. It doesn't hurt like it did a week or two ago. I'm even still anticipating some hearing eventually being restored.

It's been three weeks since my surgery. It's so hard to believe it's been that long already. I did get sprung from jail a few times in the past week. I went out to lunch last Monday and then went shopping, where I used the walker. Oh, that was horrible. I vowed to not need the walker after that, and I graduated to a cane. For twenty minutes. I'm not coordinated enough to walk with a cane. I couldn't figure out when to lean, and when to let go. I moved quickly onto hanging on to wall-and-arm status.

My first real social outing, not including going to the doctor or going for my weekly Monday lunch with Mish, was to go hear great music on Thursday night. I begged and whined a little for my friend Deb to take me, which she did while Ken was at his own music rehearsal. I might have misrepresented that Ken knew where we were going. I also didn't tell her it was my first and only, so-far, nighttime outing until we were already there. She only freaked out a little when I told her. We only stayed a short while, and Ken got home before we did. He was a little annoyed with me for not telling him where we were going and was very glad nothing happened.

I went for a really long walk last Friday ... well, it seemed really long since it was truly my first walk post surgery with Mish ... about a mile round trip. Took me FOREVER! I had lots of energy for the whole walk, and at the end I was pretty tired. We stopped and had tea, which was nice, and then when I got home, I was filled with excited energy and didn't nap at all and stayed up until 1:00 AM working on a project. That was a big mistake.

I woke up tired Sunday and went to the Unitarian Church where we are members, where I used the wall to hold me up as my friends greeted me. I am noticing I am more unstable when there are a lot of people and distractions around. I'm okay with a small group target, but too many people at once is more than my addled brain can handle right now. And then that afternoon, there was another matinee at another local community theater. By the end of the show, I just wanted to crawl into bed, so I didn't even congratulate the cast. I NEVER do that ... but these are strange times, right?

Today was better. Monday lunch, followed by PT. I'm dizzier than I was two months ago, but not as dizzy as I could be. I am walking alone (without an arm or a wall) occasionally, as long as I can focus my sight on something not moving. I sometimes feel like I could even drive my car. But I promised to wait and see what the docs say next Thursday at my follow-up appointment.

I know I have to set better boundaries and learn the difference between pushing myself and doing too much.

Until then I'll just have to take my own advice. Have patience.

COMMENTS

NANCY said: As my surgery professor used to say, "Little drops of water, little grains of sand, make the mighty ocean and the mighty land." I'm thinking that "slowly," as in, "take it slowly," is not in your vocabulary.

In response to realizing I lied by omission.

DEB said: Yeah ... only freaked out a little ... riiiiight.

My response: He was never mad at you for a moment, I was "in trouble" for slipping out, even with an escort.

JACQUI said: Step by step, inch by inch, slowly she turned ... Gotta love Lucille Ball.

DUDLEY said: Step by step, day by day, perseverance furthers being peace being alive.

TARA said: I have been using what I learned as the family member of a patient in being a better nurse. I am glad none of your helpers have let you fall ... love you, Nurse Ratched ... p.s. not enough Tiki-Man exercises on your daily schedule.

———

March 5, 2010: Walking and talking

I am coming up on my one-month anniversary of my surgery. When I look back at the days just before February 10, I remember how absolutely petrified I was ... of all the possible surgery outcomes: paralysis, stroke, incontinence, depression, confusion. I had complete faith and confidence in my doctors; I just didn't know what I couldn't know ... how my body and brain would react to the trauma of surgery. And I didn't know what my needs would be when I got home. Thankfully, Mish and Ken had lined up friends who would be with me 24/7 just in case I needed something—anything—and just in case I was less abled than I needed to be to take care of myself.

It seems like no one expected me to be this far along this quickly. Even though there were hundreds of messages to the contrary—"You are so strong," " You will walk and be fine," " I know the results will be good"—when people saw me the first week after my surgery, they were surprised and shocked how I looked and how well I was getting around. Now it's more than three weeks, and I am happy to say that I have graduated to "care free," in that I get to be alone in my house!

Now you might not think it is such a big deal to be alone, but to me it means that I am no longer considered a "fall risk" by my family and that everyone can relax about my potential to faint on cue. I promise to not do stupid or potentially dangerous things like water ski or mow the lawn or do laundry (thank you Dr. Wonderful for that permission slip). The "jailers," as I have been referring to them (in jest, I so appreciate each and every one of the friends who sit, walk, talk, laugh, listen, practice my exercises, share, and keep me company so that time passes faster), will still be on phone standby if I need to go somewhere like a PT appointment, or "just in case" something happens. I don't expect an "in case" will come up.

I have yet to brainstorm the perfect thank you for each of these people. I don't know if I will ever be able to thank them enough for these past three weeks.

I am scheduled to have a hearing test on Tuesday, and then my one-month check-in with Dr. Wonderful and Dr. Superman on Thursday. I'll find out then if I am cleared to drive, do Yoga, take other vitamin supplements, and go for acupuncture to check on my left arm weakness, which is getting better, but slowly. I know I will have to start slowly, but I am really looking forward to being more myself.

This morning, Mish and I took an hour-long walk at the waterfront. The bad news is that that same walk used to take me half as long. The good news is that this time, I walked completely without assistance. No walker. No cane. No hanging on my companion's arm. Like a big girl. I am so looking forward to getting around the lake again.

No matter how long the walk takes.

And I know it will happen soon.

———

March 11, 2010: Norman doesn't live here anymore ... twenty-nine days later ...

It's been quite a week. On Tuesday, I went to the Speech and Hearing center at Western Washington University in Bellingham WWU to have my one-month post-op hearing test. It basically flatlined. Nothing left on the left. But the tech said that my eardrum wasn't moving at all, and since I was complaining of sinus pain, there was a possibility of some sort of congestion there, and who knows what will happen once it is reduced?

But it doesn't matter to me. I was not expecting to retain any hearing on my left side ... it's all Dr. Superman's desire to place another feather in his cap to have another patient walk away from this surgery with some residual hearing. I'm good either way.

Wednesday I had my second post-op PT. Because of the middle ear congestion, I was having trouble walking backward, heel to toe. Okay, maybe it wasn't the congestion. You try it. Can you do that easily? I did have balance trouble just standing heel to toe, eyes open, so I know I have to work on that, but I don't feel like this is still surgery recovery. I don't think I could have done that thirty days ago either. In addition, my left/right hand coordination is off, which makes me nervous because of what I do for a living. (I type. A lot.) The last thing at PT was a yoga ball exercise. They had me sit on a yoga ball and "march" by slowly raising one leg at a time. The goal was to keep my balance when I did that. Not so much. Yeah, my inner core is totally mush. I gotta work on that too.

Today Mish took me to Seattle for my post-op appointments, and Dr. Backous said not to expect any hearing to return, that I would have had some by now. I have not yet given up, and I may not ever give up completely. But, like I said, I am good either way. In response to my questions about my left and right hand coordination issue, Dr. Farrokhi assured me that it was due to temporary bruising of the brain stem, and that by practicing and using my left hand as much as possible, it will improve in time. That was very comforting and encouraging.

Also today when I saw both surgeons, I wasn't medicated and I remembered everything that they said. I saw the post-op MRI of Norman. Or should I say, where Norman used to live. He is GONE!!! Just a dot or two remains where he used to take up residency. I ordered a copy of the MRI, so when I get it, I'll make a photo for my computer desktop ... before and after. It's amazing and such a relief to see that it's really over.

In addition to the good news about my hearing status and my lack of coordination, both doctors agreed I that can resume all of my previous activities, but to be conscious of my activity level. It may take up to a year to get my stamina back to my pre-surgery intensity. I can drive, do yoga, do Pilates, use hair products, get massages, get acupuncture, and drink (though not while I am driving.)

Tonight I plan to go out to listen to music. I was going to drive myself but decided I didn't want my first solo to be in the dark, so I am bumming a ride. It's a little unnerving to drive in the dark yet, so getting a ride is great, even though I won't be drinking anything.

Mish thinks I need to push myself more to help my stamina ... so tomorrow (late) morning we are getting back up on the horse. I am planning my first trek around Lake Padden in a month, and I cannot wait.

COMMENTS
MISH said: Boy, that Mish sounds like a real slave driver!

TARA said: Slave driver, Baby Ratched, Dr. Superman, Dr. Wonderful, Norman, caregivers ... boy, do any of us have real names? Best news ever. Love to you and all of those who have helped along the way. Thank you ... Nurse Ratched

Chapter 7. A WHOLE NEW NORMAL

March 23, 2010: A whole new normal

I am forty days post-surgery. I have resumed all my activities pre-surgery, except for laundry. I'm holding fast on that one.

I have resumed my walks, have completed the whole trek around the lake and the waterfront, done a big grocery shopping trip, made dinners, driven around town, and gone dancing a few times. I tried drinking, but I still can't tolerate the taste of wine, red or white, and the liquors I have "tested" have left me with morning headaches.

My overall stamina is getting a bit better, I am still taking as many naps a day as I can fit in, mostly because I do not sleep well at night. Though I have not slept well for years, it was not as big of a problem before. I remember in an earlier blog that I considered that Norman was the Energizer Battery in my head ... I may not have been far from the truth. Either way, I am more tired now and hope that it will dissipate in the future and that I can get my old energy level back. I've been advised it may take up to a year.

So you may be wondering, with my activity and energy levels in the pink, why I haven't gone back to work yet?

Let's talk about stress and its effect on the brain. This is unscientific research done with a sampling of one. (That would be me.)

Stressful situations may include but are not limited to: being around a lot of my friends or people I do not know, and/or being around people I know but do not enjoy hanging out with. They may also include dealing with deadlines and time constraints, such as having to be at a certain place at a certain time, and not being able to leave when I find myself tiring or stressed (see above). And finally, the most recently discovered stressful situation is creative/cognitive thinking on a deadline. It exhausts me, makes my head throb, and I become stupid.

The more "recovered" I feel, the more "normal" I try to be, which has inevitably brought on more stress by putting me into the aforementioned circumstances. I am trying to avoid, or at least remove myself from, the situations as I become aware of them, but sometimes that is too late.

I went to my office last week and talked to one of my bosses. She seems to be okay with me not coming back for a few more weeks. I'm not sure when her patience will wear off.

Hopefully not before my ability to deal with added stress has returned.

COMMENTS
TARA said: You need to rest and listen to your body. The last thing you need to do is overdo it and pass out.

April 7, 2010: As if nothing ever happened
I went back to work today. It seemed like it would be an easy thing to do; before my surgery I had been working part time (twenty to thirty hours a week) for the past four years, so my first day back I planned to only work four hours.

Before my surgery, I would go in at eight or nine in the morning and work until two, but sometimes stay until three or four in the afternoon without a break. I do not want that to happen anymore. Today I went in at eleven, so I was able to take my regular daily walk this morning and go home before work to get ready.

One of my two bosses was there when I arrived. I spent the first hour just getting my bearings again. My bosses are legal guardians, they ensure the personal needs and/or management of finances for people who can't do such things for themselves and don't have a family member able to do it for them.

"Things are different, more streamlined," she said.

"That's fine."

"We want you to be able to do more office management and case management kind of work."

"That's fine."

And then she told me her office email had been bouncing back from people for a week or two. Our IT guy was unable to help. I opened my desk drawer and found the file that had all the passwords to our website and our linked email and gave it to her. An hour later, she was still messing with it, so I took it back. Within the hour, I remembered, from some recesses of my brain, to go into webmail to delete the stuff off the server. (It had been almost two years since I did it the last time … my, how time flies when you are having fun.) There were more than 2500 emails clogging up her email on her server. No wonder. So now it's working again, and from that short burst of focus, I felt both a high and a spinny head.

I did it though. I was able to solve a problem, brain surgery and all. It was as if nothing ever happened.

Shortly after that, one of my favorite clients called and was shocked that I was at work. He came in a little later and was asking all kinds of questions—Was I done with treatment? Was I okay to work? How long was I in the hospital? This was not completely out of the blue, since one of the reasons he is our client is that he had a brain injury years ago.

It was strange being back, dealing with clients, fixing problems in the office. But it felt good. Like I was doing something besides just staring at my computer or TV at home.

And then I left work at three o'clock!! My boss seemed a little surprised. I suppose because I had only been there for four hours.

"You're leaving? Are you coming back?"

"Tomorrow," I said.

"Are you sure you want to?"

"Do you want me to?"

"Yes," she said.

So I went home and considered stopping for a glass of something stronger than water somewhere … anywhere … but I honestly was too exhausted to pick a place to go to. I went home and literally collapsed on my bed and fell asleep for almost an hour.

We'll take it slow.

COMMENTS

DEB said: Nothing has changed and everything has changed.

My response: Amen, Sister!

EPILOGUE

Two weeks later, I found myself in Los Angeles at my mother's bedside, as she underwent a mastectomy for a malignant tumor discovered after my surgery. Twenty-one days later, she was gone as a result of complications from that surgery. To this day, I swear my mother had made a deal with God, to let me recover fully from my surgery and to take her in my place. My mother was there for my first breath; I was blessed with being able to be there for her last.

I left my job. I was unemployed for five months.

I got a new job.

In December, 2010, we hosted our Second-Annual Last Chanukah Party.

At the one-year anniversary of my surgery, I had a new MRI. Immediately after, the three of us, Ken, Dr. Wonderful, and I, sat in the little exam room.

We talked about our kids, what I'd been doing since my surgery, about GimmeAMinute, about work.

He asked me how I was feeling, checked my smile, had me puff out my cheeks. We talked about my ear ringing, and then we all looked at the MRI together for the first time.

He was not happy.

Norman had apparently left me a little gift. A small, 3 mm

something. It was not there right after my surgery. Possibly scar tissue, possibly a new tumor. He said he would call me later with the radiologist's report.

Three hours later, he called. He started off with "I have bad news." My heart dropped. Oh my God, I thought, it's really cancer this time. Then he said, "I can't log into www.gimmeaminute.com here at the hospital; I'll have to wait until I get home."

My head gets to feeling spinny.

Then he said that the radiologist agreed with him, that he can't really tell if the tumor (little as it is) is scar tissue or new tumor, and he advised us to check again in three months and then at regular intervals.

In any case, I now will have to have regular MRIs for the rest of my natural life.

Hey, it could be worse, right?

For now, for today, I'll just believe Stacey Scar Tissue is my new BFF (Best Friend Forever).

Assuming she does not grow, she will just sit there as a constant reminder … not that that's a bad thing …

If she does grow, well, we will just cross that bridge when we come to it, won't we?

I have so many people to be grateful to for the support, encouragement, and kind words during all this time.

I've gained self-reliance, I gained deeper connections with friends and family. Ken lost his dad, I lost my mom.

I'm feeling physically okay. I'm still wondering when I'll be able to jump up and down (literally) and land on both feet at once. My surgeon told me that whatever I am having trouble doing, I should do more of to improve my ability to do it. Even if I look funny? I'm still not up to the trampoline, but I'm thinking about working on it.

I started a new bucket list. This book was on it. I want to be able to be there for someone, anyone, just like Adrienne, Cheryl, and Adam were there for me.

I am very clear about my boundaries, and I am no longer blinded by my desire to be "all that and a bag of chips."

The lemonade we have made out of lemons here at home is refreshing and remarkable. We take things one day at a time and appreciate each other more than ever. My siblings and I are dealing with our loss in different ways in different stages, and I miss my mom so much every day. I am trying to keep making her proud, and I will always remember how much she loved and appreciated my friends for being there for me when she could not be.

So where are we now? I can tell you where I am. I am here. To stay.

I still have loud ringing in my left ear. Which is the only thing I can "hear" on that side. I don't like to be teased about it when I am tired. I also don't like to be snuck up upon on that side. It's not funny. I can only have one conversation at a time. If I am on the phone, don't even bother asking me to say hi to the person on the phone for you. Unless you write me a note, it's not happening.

I can't walk well in the dark. I need to see to balance.

I can't walk backwards and talk to someone. Maybe that's not smart anyway.

When I'm really, really tired, parts of my face start to tingle, like it's just recovering from the dentist's Novocain wearing off. But it never feels like that when I wake up.

I have a positive outlook on life. I have a positive attitude about discovering, deciding, and doing what's important. Like the way my priorities changed when I had children, they renewed on February 10, 2010. I care about things that are important, like relationships with my family and friends. I am aware I cannot be all things to all people, I can only do what I can do, and I continue to pay attention to my limits of overstretch.

I say "no" as much, if not more, than I say "yes."

To be honest, I wasn't sure I could learn anything new again. The occasional thought of failing freaks me out. I am fearful I will forget things, important things. Instead of focusing on the crucial information, in the past, I junked up my head with minutiae. Yeah, it's been a learning process all over.

I live every day, one day at a time. I plan my days ahead. I am six months out, and it is filling fast. There are milestones ahead, and I will savor every second of them. And I will be present.

A recent horoscope told me to not look back to my past, and while I understand that conceptually, I realize that I need to be mindful of how I got here. I am a true believer in quantum theory, and I know I didn't get here alone. I was never alone. Don't you think for one minute I am not grateful for the help, support, encouragement, and love I received from family, friends, and strangers.

I am keeping that gratitude energy going. I smile at the smallest provocation. And sometimes, when I smile, it reminds me of where I was not so long ago, and I think of my supporters.

Look at all the things that have happened in the world, in the country, in the state, in town, at home, in a life ...

In terms of a newborn (let's not even start with the whole gestational piece), the ability to come from nothing but a living, breathing, eating creature, to being able to communicate, respond to stimuli, make decisions, to move from one place to another, to roll, crawl, and sometimes even walk without assistance, all can develop over the course of that first year.

One year.

For clarification purposes, the Days of Norman's Existence, or "DONE," defines the period in my life from the date of Norman's discovery until the date of his extraction. Only six months, but still, a period to acknowledge and respect.

DONE and done. I found myself at a place I would not wish on anyone, and if I had to do it all again, I would definitely do it. I don't mean just the surgery, but being DONE really taught me so much about living fully.

And now that DONE is done, my perspective on life still remains the same ... I'm living in the moment. What's different is that I'm looking forward to a future. I don't think I would have been able to say that a year ago. I mean, I said it after I woke up from surgery, but as much as I knew I chose the right doctors, you just never know, you know?

I followed the Kathi Goertzen story ... she was the brilliant Seattle newscaster who had a tumor not too different from mine, but hers kept growing back. One of her final surgeries nicked her facial nerve. When I first saw her in a photo after that, I was shocked and saddened, and then I watched a video report as she headed into yet another surgery.

Truth is, the more she talked, the less visually apparent her nerve damage was, and her true beauty showed through. I guess I got used to how she looked, and so I didn't notice after a few minutes. She knew that she'd never get back to doing news until her nerve completely regenerated, as the damage also affected her speech. It's society's bias against the less-than-perfect. I prayed for her. She never got her old life back; she passed away in August of 2012.

There but for the grace of God ...

March 27, 2013 Norman 0 for 3

Today is the day of my three-year post surgery MRI and check up. Dr. Wonderful is going over my MRI, and as I peer over his shoulder, I see that Stacey Scar Tissue has morphed into something that pours over into about two thirds of the left side of my brain. "Don't worry," he says with a smile. "I sucked all of the new tumor out with a turkey baster."

I wake up with a start. Only a dream, I tell myself. Breathing. I'm so anxious I am sure my blood pressure is over the charts.

I drive to Seattle by myself. It's the first time in over three years I have done any part of my journey, except for write, by myself. Without a second full set of ears. I decide I had been babying myself too long, and I should get over it and get on with it. Yep. Then I had that dream and got scared all over again.

I'm not complaining, and I'm reminding myself daily that my tumor is not and never was cancer, but I'm thinking about my multiple falls in the past six months. Is it indicative of new growth, my lack of core balance, or something else? Something simple? Something worse? Am I enough of a drama queen?

I try to connect with friends who live in Seattle as I make my drive down, both to kill time and distract myself before my appointment. One was working, and one was, ironically enough, back in Whatcom County where I live and would be heading back to Seattle before I returned home. I end up getting to my MRI appointment an hour early, but luckily, they are able to take me in a little early—a good thing since it was a LOOONNNNGGG MRI. Why is it that when you are having your ears and brain checked, they put you in a really noisy machine for about an hour? Good thing I don't have a headache!

When the MRI is done, I go to wait for my appointment with Dr. Wonderful. He is running "on time," which means I get to wait, and wonder, and worry about whether my dream will come true. His familiar comforting face when he walks into the exam room makes me think he'd be really good at poker or talking to small children about the tooth fairy. I can never tell what he's thinking. He looks at the scans, and with no difference in demeanor—happy, excited, or not so much—he tells me the pictures are exactly the same, if not a teensy weensy bit smaller than last year, and that I can safely take a year off and come back for a re-scan in two years.

I ask him if I can be on the five-year plan.

Silence.

"Um," Dr. Wonderful started (this guy NEVER says "um"), "I'm not really comfortable with that. Would you rather go to get your MRI in Bellingham? Is it the expense? Is it the drive down here? I can call you if there are any changes."

I assured him it was not the drive to Seattle—I have insurance, thank God, and my husband's gainful employment. I assured him it was nothing personal. I like seeing him, I said, but I'd rather come down and have coffee or lunch with him. He's a nice guy; he has great stories about his kids, who I'm sure I have funded to put through college at this point.

"I just want all of this behind me," I said. Like any surgery to correct a broken, torn, infected body part, at some point it just becomes part of your backstory. Right?

Again silence. For a second

"How about this. Come back in two years, and if all is the same as today, we'll go to the five-year plan. How does that sound?"

Like I'm about to get my life back to normal.

ACKNOWLEDGMENTS

I did not travel this journey alone. To all of the wonderful physicians, medical staff, and caregivers, especially Farrokh Farrokhi, MD, Paula L. Brown, LAC, Dr. Woody Bernard, Douglas D. Backous, MD, and Ann Knowles, MD. Tara, Mish, Nancy, Alyssa, Barbara, Francie, Marsha, Ro, Dudley, Jill, and Deb have been more than sisters and friends. You have been my lifeboat. Zoe and Caleb, you are the shore that I was always looking toward. Ken, you are my everything—my best friend, my strongest supporter, my biggest fan, and the love of my life. In addition I must acknowledge the more than 296 family, friends, and strangers-turned-friends who followed and supported my journey via the Internet and the many supportive F.U.N. crew members. I would love to but could not possibly name all of you here. I love and appreciate all of you more than you could ever possibly know.

For more information on Acoustic Neuroma:

Acoustic Neuroma Association of the United States – www.anausa.org
Acoustic Neuroma Association of Canada – www.anac.ca

All profits from the sale of this book will be donated and divided equally between **ANAUSA** and **ANAC**

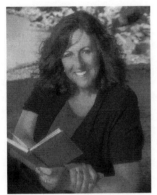

CHERYL CROOKS

ABOUT THE AUTHOR

Marla makes her home in the Pacific Northwest. She lives in Bellingham, Washington with her husband Ken. Her favorite children are
Zoe and Caleb.